NAKED AT 50

STACI BERKOVITZ

To Mom and Dad: The reason I get to tell this story is because you included me in yours. Love you.

UNTITLED

Staci Berkovitz

UNTITLED

Times I've ever been naked with a bunch of strangers?
   Zero.
   Until now. Until 50.

INTRODUCTION

My mom died at 52. She was diagnosed with pancreatic and liver cancer which was discovered during what was thought as a normal gallbladder surgery. In six weeks, she was gone. I am sure you are thinking, "What a happy way to start this book, Staci ... or should we call you Debbie Downer? Thanks for pepping me up by shoving morbid thoughts of mortality my way."

But hear me out. We are all going to die. I know, first time you have ever heard the news, but it is true. No matter our ethnicity, age, religion or shoe size, we will die at some point, and who knows how or when. If you have been on this earth for more than a few years, you have probably known somebody who is no longer here. The loss of a loved one is terribly sad (except for the people that we are happy to see go like tyrants, terrorists or people who don't put the toilet seat down). And yet, we will all be "that" loved one at some point.

So, with this piece of news, let's not worry about

how/when you are going to die. Let's focus more on **how you choose to live.**

When I began thinking about turning 50, I shuddered. Here were some of my thoughts:

That number looks old.

Like really old.

Like menopausal old.

Like white-haired old.

Like Golden Girls old.

As a fitness instructor and vibrant 49-year-old, I knew how to make life all it could be. Solo travel-check. Visit all 50 states. Yep. Boudoir photos. Three times. Swam with dolphins. Taught at Harvard (OK, it was two songs at a Harvard Zumba class, but still). I have lived abroad, ran wellness retreats, landed on a glacier in Alaska and played with monkeys in Japan. I was married and then later divorced. I adopted four children. Became a grandma. Lived life fully. Old wasn't in my vocabulary. But I imagined when the calendar changed to 5-0 on that fateful day in May, I would grab a walker and a Mumu and peace out my youthful exuberance.

I sat with that for a while, clearly not excited about it. Then I remembered my mom. Age 52. Something clicked inside me. I was indeed living the privileged life. The privilege of living. I was not going to stop living a full life just because of a few white hairs and a half-dollar birthday. Hence, an idea was born.

Naked at 50 came to me when I leaned into really deciding how I wanted to celebrate this milestone. Yes, I have had a very full life, BUT that doesn't mean the story needed to end there. No way! On the contrary, I wanted my 50th year to be celebrated trying 50 new things—big, small and in between—that I had never done before. Life does not end at 50.

And guess what, friend? My biggest joy would be if as you were reading this book, you got inspired to create your full and exuberant life by making your own list of things that light you up for whatever year/birthday that is important to you. Does it have to be 50 experiences? No! It can be one new thing a month, or one a year or one every Tuesday.

When I chose the title *Naked at 50*, I knew it was more than just a catchy phrase—it captured exactly how I felt as I stepped into that new chapter of my life. Turning 50 had felt like stripping away all the layers I'd built up over the years—the expectations, the pretenses, even some of the fears. Turning 50 was both terrifying and liberating. It wasn't just about physical changes, though that was part of it. It was about embracing who I truly was, without apology. It was about starting fresh, shedding past expectations and moving forward with an openness to whatever came next—vulnerable, raw and unapologetically me.

This book is written in three parts, and weaves together practical advice for navigating the milestone of turning 50 and living vibrantly and fully. The first part is focused on *your* reflection and discovery—looking back at all the things that got you to be the YOU of today and really creating awareness of who you are now. The second part is planning and preparation—how you can plan and embrace living life in the most vibrant, fullest, and healthiest way from 50 and beyond. The final part of the book is a walk through all 50 of the new experiences that I had during the year I turned 50. You may love or loathe the ideas. Either way, they are there to give you a springboard to your own bucket list. Among them, some may seem to be a "go big or go home" mentality, while others might be described as small and unassuming. What matters is the novelty and openness of each experience and how it helps to embrace curiosity and freshness in life. Green and growing or ripe and rotten—you choose.

Whether you're on the brink of your 50th year or simply seeking ways to make any year unforgettable, this book is here to guide and inspire you. Get ready to be informed, engaged and motivated to transform your 50th year, or any year, into a truly memorable experience. Hold my cane, let's go!

ONE

THE SIGNIFICANCE OF REFLECTION - MIRROR, MIRROR ON THE WALL LET'S TALK ABOUT IT ALL

"KNOWING YOURSELF IS THE BEGINNING OF ALL WISDOM."— ARISTOTLE

HAVE YOU EVER LOOKED BACK AT A PICTURE FROM YOUR youth and thought, "Why did I think that outfit or haircut was a good idea?" I mean, jelly shoes with leg warmers? Aerosol-winged hair (which I rocked, by the way)? Shoulder pads that could be repurposed by NFL teams. But outside of the fashion tragedies, we all have done a lot of life by the time we hit age 50. Reaching that mid-century mark (does that make you feel old when you hear the word "century"?) is a great time to consider all that has happened in the first 50 years.

During this time, it is totally normal to experience a shift in perspective, re-evaluate your goals and reassess your priorities. As a matter of fact, it is not only normal but important. When I was in sixth grade, I told everyone I wanted to be a duck trainer and a camel rider. I am

1

happy to report that my career trajectory went into a totally different direction. However, if I had stayed the course, and never reflected on what I wanted to do as I changed and grew (and went through puberty), who knows what part of the Sahara I would be hanging my camel saddle in. The same goes for first loves, choices for entertainment and en vogue phrases that were "totally gnarly."

Reflection midlife gives us a chance to really decide what we *want* life to look like now versus what it sort of evolved to be. Sometimes we evolve accidently, and sometimes, we make a conscious decision to change. So, with that said, the following pages are your nice walk down *Reflection Lane*. It is essentially an opportunity to do some really meaningful reflecting and journaling. You can use a notebook or your computer, or you can write directly in this book (unless you got it from the library— they frown upon that). Turn on some relaxing tunes, light a candle and let's get our reflection on!

Reflection on Achievements:

You don't have to have an Olympic medal or a huge home to have achieved something in life. Sometimes, we tend to be hard on ourselves and minimize what we have accomplished. Think about your life and brag, knowing that nobody has lived a perfect life. Celebrate the big and little things!

What are some things that you most proud of accomplishing by this age?

. . .

What have been some big milestones you have reached?

Are there any goals you set in your earlier years that you have accomplished?

Growth and Wisdom:

As the adage says, with age comes wisdom. Lean into what your 50-year-old self has learned versus your mindset at age 20. Love, life and loss teaches us.

Describe a significant life lesson you've learned by the age of 50. How has it shaped your life?

In what ways have you grown personally and emotionally over the years?

How do you handle challenges and setbacks now compared to when you were younger?

Re-evaluation of Priorities

Much like my sixth-grade self, wanting to be a camel rider, our ideas and what is important to us changes as we grow and get older. What was important to you in the past may have lost its luster.

Have your priorities shifted as you entered your 50s? If so, how?

. . .

What aspects of your life bring you the most joy and fulfillment?

Are there any aspects of your life that you would like to prioritize moving forward?

Relationships and Connections

Relationships change over time, and this is the normal evolution of our existence. As you dive into the next few questions, ponder how your relationships have changed.

Reflect on your relationship with family and friends. How have they evolved over the years?

Are there relationships that have become more important to you? Conversely, are there relationships that you feel the need to change?

How do you balance personal time with social connections? How do you feel about your current friendships?

Health and Wellbeing

Health is wealth. How true that is! Examine your state of health with these questions.

How would you describe your current approach to health and wellbeing? Are there areas you would like to improve?

What are some specific steps you have taken or plan to take to maintain or improve your physical and mental health?

Are you current with all your immunizations, screenings and annual exams?

Phew! How was that? Anything pop out? Any surprises? If you have seen 50 years on this earth, you have seen a few things (unless of course you come from another planet, and in that case, welcome to earth—a wonderful and beautiful mess). Sometimes looking back can provide clarity going forward. As long as we don't stay "stuck" in the narratives of what was or what should be, the past can be a great teacher.

Now it is time to get a little more specific. This next reflection activity will help you really examine those moments worth celebrating (and those other moments in which therapy was needed or is still needed). Complete these pages with a sense of love and grace for yourself, and a celebration of all that you have achieved and those things that you have overcome.

Highs of My Life:

Personal Triumphs: (Reflect on your greatest personal achievements, such as milestones, successes and moments of joy. Consider writing about things like relationships, family moments or personal growth—see your answer to the very first reflection question.)

Professional Successes: (List your proudest moments in your career, educational accomplishments, or any other professional successes that have shaped your journey.)

Memorable Experiences: (Think about the most memorable trips, adventures or experiences that brought you happiness and fulfillment.)

Lows of My Life:

Challenges and Obstacles: Reflect on the most difficult challenges you've faced. Consider personal losses, health struggles or other hardships.

Lessons Learned: For each low, think about what you learned from the experience. How did it shape you, and what did you take away from it?

• • •

Moving Forward: Consider how you've grown from your lows and what you hope to carry forward into the next chapter of your life.

Gratitude Reflection:

Write a few thoughts about what you are grateful for from the first 50 years of your life. This can include people, experiences or personal qualities that you value (notice how much space this one has-so much to be grateful for in life)!

Looking Ahead:

As you move forward, what are you most excited about? What are your hopes, dreams and goals for the next phase of your life? (If you are feeling stuck on this question, don't worry. We will dive deep into this in the next few chapters).

Now that you have completed this reflection, coupled with the last chapter's reflective look back, take some time to read the following passage aloud. No seriously. Do it. Even better if you look in the mirror while you are reading. By taking in all you reflected on above, you now have the opportunity to frame it into a healthy mindset to move forward.

Read this aloud:

"In the first 50 years of my life, the highs were

moments of tremendous personal growth and accomplishment. These milestones included [name your specific achievements or experiences], where I felt a profound sense of pride and fulfillment. These highs served as markers of my resilience, dedication and ability to overcome challenges."

"On the flip side, the lows were instances of adversity and struggle that tested my resilience. These challenges, such as [specific difficulties or setbacks], were undoubtedly tough to navigate. However, they also provided valuable lessons, highlighting my capacity for growth and adaptation in the face of adversity."

"Reflecting on both the highs and lows, I recognize that they collectively formed me and my unique experiences. The highs have been sources of joy and motivation, propelling me forward with a sense of purpose. Meanwhile, the lows have been powerful teachers, instilling in me resilience, empathy and a deeper understanding of myself."

"As I move into the next phase of my life, I carry with me the lessons and triumphs of the past 50 years. They shape my perspective, fuel my aspirations, and serve as a foundation for continued personal and emotional growth. I appreciate the richness of my life's journey and the valuable insights for the chapters yet to unfold."

TWO

THE GREAT RELEASE - LET IT GO (NOT JUST A DISNEY ANTHEM)

"IN THE PROCESS OF LETTING GO, YOU WILL LOSE MANY THINGS FROM THE PAST, BUT YOU WILL FIND YOURSELF."— DEEPAK CHOPRA

HAVE YOU EVER ATTEMPTED TO CLEAN OUT YOUR CLOSET AND found a pair of pants you swore would fit again someday? Or rifled through your bathroom cabinet only to discover ancient beauty products that have somehow outlasted your past three moves? The underwear drawer? Yeah, you're not going to see those 1998 panties on the runway anytime soon. Welcome to the world of decluttering—referred to in this chapter as the Great Release. Together, we're going to purge "stuff" and really inventory our lives. And to be clear, the "stuff" is both tangible and emotional. Yep. It's time to do some cleaning up.

Emotional Baggage (We All Have It!)

Have you ever felt the weight of holding onto emotions, experiences, or relationships that no longer serve your well-being? Much like decluttering a physical space, letting go emotionally is a journey—one that clears the way for a new chapter in your life. It's time to let that s*#t go!

I'm no therapist, but I've coached enough clients and sat with my own "stuff" to know that we carry baggage in our life "trunk" without realizing it until it shows up. When that happens, we come face to face with it, and it's not always pretty. The resentment, lingering hurt, and unrealistic expectations all contribute to a heaviness that affects our well-being. Just as you declutter your living spaces, recognizing and acknowledging this emotional load is the first step toward liberation. To quote Braveheart, "Freedommmmmmm!"

Like sorting through possessions, letting go emotionally involves a deliberate examination of experiences and relationships. Reflecting on moments that no longer contribute positively to your life allows you to discern what's worth holding onto and what needs to be released. Whether it's acknowledging that certain experiences shaped you but no longer define you, or understanding that some relationships have served their purpose, letting go becomes a conscious decision to prioritize your emotional well-being. It's leveling up—and yes, you are worth it.

Releasing emotions that no longer serve you is a powerful tool for creating space—space for personal growth, new experiences and healthier relationships. The lightness that accompanies letting go is palpable. Think of it as getting off a crowded and stuffy plane into a huge, clean, empty airport. Relief. In this newfound space, you can cultivate a more authentic version of yourself. Letting go is not just about discarding the old—it's about making room for the new and embracing the ever-evolving narrative of your life. It's time to tell a new story.

Relationships: Reason, Season, Lifetime

Let's be real. Examining the relationships in your life can be scary. Things change—jobs, illness, empty-nesting, major life events—and we change, too. Naturally, some of the relationships in your life will shift as well. That can be a hard reality to face. Avoidance may seem like the easier solution, but it won't lead to long-term peace. The good news? Like an airport, you don't have to necessarily announce your departure to everyone in your life. However, there will be some people you'll need to have tough conversations with, some that you may want to let go of, and others you'll want to invest more time and attention in moving forward. Examining relationships is difficult, but freeing. It helps to think of relationships as one of the following: a reason, a season or a lifetime.

First up, the "reason" relationships—these are the individuals who waltz in with purpose, perhaps to teach you a lesson, fill a need, offer support during a challenging time or simply share a laugh. It could be that person at work who kept everyone afloat with humor, or that friend who introduced you to EDM or your local

Bible study (different experiences, but a thumping good time at each one).

Many people in our lives are positive "reasons." It could be a teacher who inspired you, a co-worker who helped you through a tough job or a teammate who cheered you on during a softball season. You came into each other's lives for a reason, and maybe that brief assignment has been completed.

Next are the "season" relationships—those people who share a substantial part of your life's narrative. These could be college friends, work colleagues or longer romantic relationships.

Understanding the meaning behind a relationship can bring peace, especially when it ends. For example, I once dated someone who was emotionally abusive (I'm OK folks, lots of therapy and self-exploration helped me heal that one). Now, with distance, I can see that the relationship taught me about self-worth and how to recognize red flags early on. I bless and release this person, grateful for the growth.

Many of our "season" friends play positive roles in our lives. Over the span of 50 years, there are people who've come into our lives and stayed longer than the "reason" ones, but as life changes, so do these relationships. This could be the parents of your kid's soccer teammates whom you adored, but as soccer ended, so did the relationships. Or the co-worker who became a confidant but drifted apart after job changes. Each person entered your life for a reason, leaving positive imprints.

Finally, we have the "lifetime" relationships—those

who stay with you through thick and thin. These are the characters who've earned a permanent spot in your life, playing integral roles in your ongoing story. Sorting through these connections is a cherished, nostalgic journey. In my case, these are friends I've had for 30+ years, and of course, close family relationships.

Sifting through relationships isn't about dismissing people; it's about acknowledging the ebb and flow of connections. It's about recognizing when a character's role has been fulfilled and when it's time for a new subplot to unfold. Letting go doesn't erase memories; it makes space for the evolution of your story. I once read that we have sacred contracts with people before coming to Earth, and when a relationship ends, it's like that contract has been fulfilled. Thank the person for the lessons they brought into your life.

Remember, it's not about the quantity of connections but the quality of the roles they play. As you stand in these cleared spaces, you're not just tidying up your social circle; you're deciding who you want by your side moving forward.

Action Time:

First, make a list of people in your life who you feel connected with in positive ways. These are people you feel your best around.

What are ways that you can nourish these relationships?

. . .

Once you make that list, consider who is NOT on it. What relationships do you need to kindly let go?

Who of those people do you value enough to stay connected to for this next chapter of life? Who is coming to the next decade with you? Give yourself the grace to let in those who you want by your side and to let go of those who you don't in the most loving way possible.

Releasing the Stories and Narratives That No Longer Serve You

We tell ourselves stories for years until, in our minds, they become the only truth that exists. After a while, these stories start to define us and, at times, can become our own prison.

The outdated narratives—the antique stories that may have once held significance—have lost their relevance. Yet, sometimes, we hold onto them too tightly when it's time to let go. Much like flipping through an old family album and realizing that some stories have yellowed with time, these narratives have aged. Perhaps you've been a people pleaser or perfectionist all your life (guilty!), and by doing so, you felt that's where your value and worth come from. As adults, we understand we were raised by imperfect people, just as we are imperfect now. So, it's time to move past others' expectations of you. As you declutter these antiquated tales, you make space for a mental attic filled with narratives that align with the present version of yourself.

Now, let's talk about the not-so-nice stories we tell

about (gulp) ourselves—the villainous monologues that undermine our self-worth, resilience, or potential. These narratives are like characters attempting a hostile takeover of your mental screenplay. Maybe you've heard some of these phrases before: *Who are you kidding? You're not as smart or capable as your colleagues. You're too fat/skinny/ugly/tall/short/ordinary for whatever you want to do.*

Sorting through these toxic tales is like editing a script, removing lines that no longer contribute to the plot. Release these damaging stories. It isn't always easy, as they may have once served a purpose—perhaps by keeping you safe or sane. Maybe they helped you survive situations that felt too difficult to face at the time. But now, it's time to let them go and make room for a mental storyline that empowers and uplifts.

Become your own best cheerleader. One habit I adopted years ago is thanking my "yesterday self." For example, if I find Tylenol in my purse when I have a headache, I silently say, *"Thank you, Yesterday Staci, for putting that in there."* It's about recognizing the same goodness and appreciation we give to others and allowing ourselves to be part of that gratitude party.

Lastly, we face the irrelevant narratives—the unfinished ideas and goals that we were going to do "one day." These are the stories that may have started with potential but no longer contribute to the evolving plot of your life. Letting go of these incomplete tales is like closing a book to make room for a new chapter. These often start with a lot of "I should have..." It might sound like, *"I should have become a doctor,"* or, *"I shouldn't have dated so-and-so."* Stop "shoulding" on yourself. You're here today. You're alive. You get to toss the stories that don't go anywhere. As you release these narratives, you create a mental library filled with stories that resonate with your current journey.

You did it! You created space in your mental and emotional world. That is pretty bad-ass and not an easy feat. Take a few deep breaths. Give yourself a hug. Now, it is time to focus on the physical stuff in which we need to determine the value it has (or doesn't have) in this stage of your life.

Letting go of "Stuff"

Phew. That got serious. How are you doing after the emotional release? Really though, letting go of the emotional stuff is just as important as the physical. The inside always encourages change on the outside. So, with that thought, we are going shift into material things and really decide which of your things have earned a place to stay with you or if it is time to set it free.

When my mom passed away, we had to go through all of her things at her apartment. I will never forget the endless stacks of clothes, books, papers, etc. The "stuff" got to stay, but she didn't. We donated almost everything. Getting rid of things is a gift to both yourself to make room for the new and a gift for those who will remain once you are no longer here. Put on your sorting hat, and let's dive in to letting go.

The Closet

Starting with the simplest category – clothes and your

closet—a treasure trove of memories, outdated fashion and well-worn shoes. As you sort through the garments that once held sentimental value (surely that Espirit fluorescent jacket will make a comeback, right?) it is time to really look at each piece of clothing and ask, do I want to take this with me in this next chapter of life? Because once you let it go, you will have created space. Sit with that feeling for a minute. Space. With space comes the ability to grow. Doesn't that feel good? Besides, do you really need the glitter mini-skirt or the suit you wore to your third cousin's wedding? If it doesn't make you feel fantastic (or incredibly comfortable) wearing it, usher it out.

Now, it is time to do the same with your undergarments: Underwear, bras, socks, ties, etc. (Hint: If it has holes in it, it is time to say goodbye).

Action Time:

In the spirit of Marie Kondo, create three piles: **Keep, Donate, and Discard**. Touch each item. Thank it for its service. And ask yourself, "Does this item fit the life I'm stepping into?" If not, it's time for it to find a new home.

The Bathroom Cabinet

Next up on the decluttering hitlist: the bathroom cabinet, a collection of expired beauty products, half-empty bottles, and forgotten remedies that have probably been around since your first college date. As you wade through this concoction of potions and elixirs, it may feel like you are on a mystical journey where you might stumble upon the fountain of youth or, at the very least, a face mask that promises to turn back time (spoiler alert: it won't).

You're not just cleaning out a cabinet; you're conducting a beauty product intervention. Those half-used bottles staring back at you like disappointed parents? Time to bid them farewell. Expired creams and lotions? Well, let's just say even they have given up hope.

As the clutter gets evicted, behold the transformation! The once chaotic cabinet is a sanctuary of self-care, a haven where your face masks can breathe, and your moisturizers can finally stop judging each other. It's not just a physical cleanse; it's a commitment to your well-being that even your facial scrubs can't help but applaud —silent cheers in the language of skincare. Ask yourself, "If I had to pack my personal care items for a trip, what would I most want and use?" That is a good indicator of what gets to stay.

As we age, our bodies change. The collection of beauty products that once worked like a champ at 40 may not be the same at 50. So, release what doesn't make you feel like your most gorgeous self. And as you do, you can't help but feel a little lighter, a little more radiant, and perhaps just a tad bit wiser about your next impulse purchase in the cosmetics aisle.

Action Time:

Yep, keep, donate and discard! You got this, Gorgeous!

Books, Papers, Knick Knacks

True story. As a health and wellness coach, I have coached and helped people through various life bumps: Weight loss, stress and anxiety, high blood pressure to name a few. I have also coached somebody how to get rid of piles and stacks of papers—enough to supply confetti for the Superbowl victor. The relief it brought this person to let go was astounding, and I subsequently did a paper purge myself after that (recycled!). So, with that said, let's dive into the next step of decluttering: the bookshelves, the paper stacks, and the kingdom of knick-knacks!

I love a good book. I have purchased many (many!) over the years. A few years ago, when I moved from my large house into a townhome, I had to give away hundreds of books. It pained me so! And then I realized, they were just collecting space. There are very few books that I read more than once. So, I had to make a conscious choice to get (most) books from the library moving forward. I do cave a few times a year and buy a new one, but I have scaled way back. Oh, this book you are reading right now, *great purchase!*

What do your bookshelves look like? Maybe there is a collection ranging from the inspiring to the utterly perplexing. Sorting through this papery jungle, you may rediscover that novel you vowed to read three summers ago—the one that doubled as a makeshift coaster for your coffee. And fear not; the textbooks from that one college class you took and never opened? They're probably discussing philosophical concepts no longer relevant since the Bush administration (the first one).

Action Time:

Go through EVERY book (yes, every single one) and decide if it is a keep, donate or discard.

Next up, paperwork clutter—a seemingly

insurmountable mountain of forgotten to-do lists, mysterious receipts, and notes from meetings that felt like secret society gatherings.

Some papers to hang on to if you do not have electronic easy access versions: Taxes for past five years, vaccines for you and the family.

Hang on to these in a safe place (safe or binder): Marriage Certificate, Divorce Decree, Birth Certificate(s), your will.

Action Time:

Keep, donate, discard (make sure to shred any documents containing important information, account numbers, etc.).

Lastly, we venture into the realm of knick-knacks—the quirky and often perplexing inhabitants of your living space. Having a five-year-old granddaughter in my house, I swear those knick-knacks multiply in the night. From miniature figurines to a huge stuffed animal collection of trips to both the Dollar Tree and Galveston, each knick-knack tells a tale of impulsive purchases and well-intentioned gifts. Don't get me started about the junk drawer (amiright?)

You might encounter relics from vacations that you only vaguely remember, or trinkets that once held sentimental value but have since been overshadowed by the march of time. It's a fun journey of rediscovery as you make decisions about what stays and what bids a fond farewell. Like it but don't love it? Take a picture and let it go.

The act of purging is not just about reclaiming

physical space; it's a declaration of your evolving identity. As the dust settles and the knick-knack kingdom is streamlined, your living space transforms into a curated gallery—a showcase of meaningful artifacts, each with a story worth telling. This is YOUR space. What really deserves a spot in this next decade?

Action Time:

Keep, donate, discard.

Now, what remains is not just an organized space but a narrative of intentional living. The decluttered shelves, cleared desk and streamlined knick-knacks are not merely a physical shift but a testament to your commitment to a life that prioritizes meaningful experiences and purposeful possessions. Look around your home. Does it match the life you are wanting to create in this next chapter? If not, remove it and anything else that feels like it no longer has a place and donate it to charity. Thank you for your service, spatula #14.

A Look into Your Habits

Now, let's shine a spotlight on your daily habits, the unsung heroes or villains (depending on the day) that shape your routine. What stays and what goes? Let's dive in.

Food

Any time I would visit my dad who lives in another state, I would go through his fridge to discard pickles that expired 10 years ago or a variety of very old condiments that witnessed the Clinton years. I was doing the good deed of purging these items for him. It wasn't until I did my own purge that I realized that the apple doesn't fall far from the tree (take my six-years expired vitamins for example). Going through your pantry and your medicine cabinet will be a life-changing experience.

Now, you may be thinking, what does the kitchen pantry and the medicine cabinet have to do with habits? One word: Health.

Your eating habits are the first stop. Go into it with a spirit of gratitude and generosity for both you and others. Then ask yourself the following: What foods do I enjoy? How do I feel after eating these foods? Will these foods help me make a commitment to prioritizing my health? There are many food pantries that would love to have what you don't want, so consider donating that food to them. Make sure to check expiration dates on food. Nobody wants to eat a moldy pickle.

Action Item:

Trigger warning: If you have experienced any type of disordered eating of any kind, only do this if you are in a good place emotionally.

Keep, donate, discard. And if there are food items that have not expired that you no longer want, consider passing these on to a local food pantry.

Medication

The medicine cabinet is an interesting place. You never know when you will need back cream or Tylenol or deworming pills. Consider your current and most common needs.

Action Item:

While "keep" is self-explanatory, donating and discarding medication is different from getting rid of a pair of socks. Check expiration dates, and make sure to dispose of medicine correctly (CVS has safe ways to do so if you are here in the U.S.).

Sleep

Next, let's dive into the habit of sleep—the mysterious, often elusive partner in your nightly escapades. Sorting through your sleep routine is like detective work. That late-night scrolling habit? It's time for an intervention. The worn-out pillow that's been with you through thick and thin? Maybe it's time to bid adieu. The act of purging transforms your bedroom into a sanctuary of rest, signaling a commitment to prioritize your well-deserved zzz's. It's not just about organizing your bedtime routine; it's about creating a sleep haven where dreams are welcomed and not rudely interrupted by endless screen time.

Look around your bedroom. Does it evoke a restful/peaceful place? Now, lay on your bed. How's the mattress? Does it need to be rotated? Replaced? How about the pillows? Sheets? Blanket? Really feel into these things and decide if they stay or go. Do you sleep better with the TV in your room, or does it keep you up at night? Would it be better somewhere else? Can you consider plugging your phone in a different room at bedtime? What temperature do you sleep best at? Play around with this until you find that sweet spot. Ceiling fan on or off? Blackout curtains on windows or do you enjoy the light coming in? Sound machine, music or silence? Sleep alone or with a partner (it is now becoming in vogue to have separate rooms to sleep in when snoring or schedules effect sleep). See all the ways you can change up sleep time?

If you are a woman and are going through peri-menopause or menopause, you may be experiencing a frequent amount of sleep disturbance, night sweats and hot flashes that significantly affect your sleep quality. Speak to your doctor about ways to help with this (and may I suggest, do a little search for OBGYN FEMALE doctors who specialize in this very thing at menopause.org).

Action Time:

The importance of sleep is no joke. As a health coach, I have seen all other things fall in life when sleep and stress are out of whack. I have struggled with getting enough quality sleep, and it is a huge determinant in all areas of life. Prioritize these two items. Use the above questions to help you make any changes to improve your sleep.

The Habits That Maybe You Don't Want to Talk About

Lastly, let's tackle the habits that might involve a glass or two or maybe even a puff. Sorting through alcohol and smoking habits is a difficult time of reckoning. Those half-empty wine bottles and lonely cigarette packs? It's time to usher them out. The act of purging transforms your recreational choices, which is a commitment to a healthier lifestyle. It's not just about breaking habits; it's about rewriting the script for a more vibrant, smoke-free and sober chapter in your life. There are so many ways to get support for this nowadays, a little Google search, find one that you feel would help you most. As you step into the next part of your life, invite the healthiest part of you to join the journey. You are worth it.

You did it! You released what no longer serves you. In its place are now blank pages in your book to write your next chapters. Ready to be the author of your intentional life?

THREE

THE INTENTIONAL YEAR - PLANNING WORLD DOMINATION (OR JUST A REALLY GOOD YEAR)

"THE SECRET OF CHANGE IS TO FOCUS ALL OF YOUR ENERGY NOT ON FIGHTING THE OLD, BUT ON BUILDING THE NEW." — SOCRATES

IF YOU'VE EVER FELT LIKE TIME IS SLIPPING THROUGH YOUR fingers (cue Abba) or like you're just along for the ride in your own life, then you're in the perfect place. We're diving into where we shift from merely celebrating a milestone to consciously creating a year that truly resonates with who you are and who you aspire to be. So, let's set the stage for your "Year of Purpose." We will define intentionality and why it matters at 50, how to set intentions that align with your core values, and craft an intentional action plan for your year ahead. This is fun stuff—you are deciding on what s%$# you want to make happen!

Intentionality

At its core, intentionality means acting with purpose and clarity. As we approach or enter our 50s, we've gathered enough life experience to know that it's not just about doing things but doing the right things—the things that light us up, that contribute to our legacy, and that align with our most profound truths." The quote "Live less out of habit and more out of intent" by Amy Rubin Flett is what we are going for with at the essence of an intentional life. It's about breaking free from habitual reactions and consciously choosing our path. In essence, it's our own awakening.

Setting Your Intentions

Intentions are not goals; they are the essence of how you want to be in the world. To set your intentions, explore your core values with questions that help you dig deep and identify what is truly important to you. Ask yourself, 'What matters most to me?' 'How do I want to feel?' 'What experiences do I wish to have?' These aren't quick questions; they require your heartfelt contemplation so take your time on really evaluating your answers.

You will be doing some self-reflection activities, including a values quiz and a strength-finder quiz. These are to help you fine-tune where you are at today (versus, say, at age 30). There are many quizzes out there on the web. If you want to dive deeper into those, do a search for: Enneagram Quiz, 16 Personalities Quiz, and Human Design Quiz to name a few. For now, we will focus on two: Values and Strengths.

Values Identification Quiz:

28

Instructions: For each statement, rate how important it is to you on a scale of 1 to 5, where 1 is "Not Important" and 5 is "Very Important." Dive into what is important to you.

1. Family: - My family's well-being and happiness are a top priority for me.

1 2 3 4 5

2. Career Success: - Achieving success and advancement in my career is important to me.

1 2 3 4 5

3. Health and Wellness: - Maintaining good physical and mental health is a priority in my life.

1 2 3 4 5

4. Financial Stability: - Having financial security and stability is crucial for my peace of mind.

1 2 3 4 5

5. Personal Growth: - Continuously learning and growing as an individual is a key aspect of my life.

1 2 3 4 5

6. Friendships: - Nurturing and maintaining meaningful friendships is important to me.

1 2 3 4 5

7. Adventure and Exploration: - Seeking new experiences and adventures is a vital part of my life.

1 2 3 4 5

8. Creativity: - Expressing myself through creative pursuits is a significant aspect of my life.

1 2 3 4 5

9. Social Justice: - Advocating for and contributing to social justice causes is important to me.

1 2 3 4 5

10. Spirituality: - Exploring and nurturing my spiritual beliefs is a fundamental part of my life.

1 2 3 4 5

11. Community Involvement: - Being actively involved in my community and making a positive impact is important to me.

1 2 3 4 5

12. Independence: - Maintaining a sense of independence and autonomy is crucial for me.

1 2 3 4 5

Values Scoring Key:

Look at the categories where you scored the highest. Consider the top 3-4 values that resonate most with you. Reflect on how these values align with your current life choices and decisions. Use these insights to guide your future actions and priorities. When you know and understand your values, you can find others who share those values as well. Like attracts like (and light attracts light).

Holistic Strengths Finder Quiz

Instructions: For each statement, rate how accurately it describes you on a scale of 1 to 5, where 1 is "Not at all like me" and 5 is "Exactly like me." Be honest with your responses.

1. Adaptability: - I am comfortable adapting to new situations and changes.

1 2 3 4 5

2. Creativity: - I enjoy coming up with new ideas and solutions.

1 2 3 4 5

3. Communication: - I am effective in expressing my thoughts and ideas to others.

1 2 3 4 5

4. Leadership: - I naturally take on leadership roles and enjoy guiding others.

1 2 3 4 5

5. Analytical Thinking: - I excel at analyzing information and making data-driven decisions.

1 2 3 4 5

6. Empathy: - I easily understand and connect with the feelings of others.

1 2 3 4 5

7. Organization: - I am skilled at organizing tasks and managing my time effectively.

1 2 3 4 5

8. Problem-Solving: - I enjoy finding solutions to challenges and overcoming obstacles.

1 2 3 4 5

9. Team Collaboration: - I work well in a team and value collaborative efforts.

1 2 3 4 5

10. Resilience: - I bounce back quickly from setbacks and challenges.

1 2 3 4 5

11. Detail-Oriented: - I pay close attention to details and ensure accuracy in my work.

1 2 3 4 5

12. Innovation: - I am open to trying new approaches and embracing innovation.

1 2 3 4 5

13. Decision-Making: - I am confident and effective in making decisions, even in challenging situations.

1 2 3 4 5

14. Networking: - Building/maintaining relationships is a strength of mine in both personal/professional spheres.

1 2 3 4 5

15. Negotiation Skills: - I am skilled at negotiating and finding win-win solutions in various life situations.

1 2 3 4 5

16. Project Management: - I excel at planning, organizing, and overseeing projects, whether at work or in personal endeavors.

1 2 3 4 5

17. Conflict Resolution: - I am effective in resolving conflicts and fostering positive outcomes in different areas of life.

1 2 3 4 5

18. Initiative: - I am proactive and take the initiative to get things done, both professionally and personally.

1 2 3 4 5

19. Attention to Other's Needs: - I prioritize and meet the needs of others effectively, whether in customer service or personal relationships.

1 2 3 4 5

20. Continuous Learning: - I actively seek opportunities for learning and personal development in various aspects of life.

1 2 3 4 5

Strengths Scoring Key:

Consider how the strengths in which you scored the highest align with different aspects of your life. Leverage these strengths holistically for increased success and fulfillment. Use this insight to guide your choices and personal development efforts in all areas of life.

Now that you have explored some of your values and strengths, let's identify what your quote or motto can be to lead your intentions (and don't worry-you don't have to get a tattoo with your motto on your right arm). Finding a quote or motto that resonates with you at the age of 50 can be a meaningful and reflective process. If you don't know where to start, use these guiding prompts: Here are some directions to help you discover your quote or motto:

- **Reflect on Your Journey:** Take some time to reflect on your life journey so far. Consider the significant experiences, challenges, achievements and lessons you've learned.
- **Identify Core Values:** Identify your core values. What principles have been guiding you throughout your life? Consider values related to family, career, personal growth, relationships and overall well-being.
- **Consider Current Priorities:** Think about your current priorities and goals. What matters most to you at this stage in your life? This could include relationships, health, personal fulfillment or giving back to the community.

- **Explore Inspirational Quotes:** Explore a variety of inspirational quotes and mottos. Look for quotes from philosophers, authors, spiritual leaders or individuals who inspire you. Consider quotes that align with your values and resonate with your current life situation.
- **Seek Inspiration in Literature and Art:** Explore literature, poetry and art for inspiration. Sometimes, a powerful line from a book, poem or artwork can encapsulate the essence of what you're feeling or seeking.
- **Connect with Personal Mantras:** Consider any personal mantras or affirmations you may have developed over the years. If you don't have one, think about what positive affirmations could serve as guiding principles for your future.
- **Ask for Input:** Reach out to friends, family or mentors for their input. Sometimes, those close to you can provide valuable insights and suggest quotes that resonate with your character and experiences.
- **Journaling:** Spend some time journaling about your feelings, aspirations and reflections. Write freely about what comes to mind, and you may discover phrases or sentiments that hold significant meaning.
- **Mindfulness and Meditation:** Engage in mindfulness or meditation practices to quiet the

mind and allow for introspection. Sometimes, moments of stillness can bring forth insights and clarity.

- **Create Your Own:** If you can't find the perfect quote, consider creating your own. Express your thoughts and feelings in a concise and impactful manner that reflects your beliefs and aspirations.
- **Test the Resonance:** Once you've identified a few candidate quotes or mottos, test their resonance. Say them out loud, write them down, and see how they make you feel. Choose the one that truly resonates with your heart and soul (OK, fine, if you want to get it as a tattoo, go for it! This is your big year!)
- **Embrace Evolution:** Remember that your quote or motto may evolve over time. Embrace the idea that as you grow and experience new phases of life, your guiding words may adapt to reflect your evolving self.

Finding your quote or motto is a personal and introspective journey. Allow yourself the time and space to explore different options until you find the one that really aligns with your values, aspirations and the essence of your life at 50. Now post it somewhere. Throw it on a sticky note. Have someone make a plaque with it. And OK, if you really want that tattoo, get it! The point is, let it be a reminder of your intention and how you are committing to live your life.

Your intentional year is combining your values, strength and motto to focus in on what really matters to you. In the next chapter, we will delve into creating a visual reminder of who we are, who we want to become, and what lights us up along the way.

FOUR
YOUR VISION BOARD - PASTING DREAMS SANS GLITTER

"CREATE THE HIGHEST, GRANDEST VISION POSSIBLE FOR YOUR LIFE, BECAUSE YOU BECOME WHAT YOU BELIEVE." — OPRAH WINFREY

THEY SAY A PICTURE IS WORTH A THOUSAND WORDS, SO imagine what a vision board has to say! It's not just a random collage of pretty images. Oh no, a vision board is like a visual GPS for your dreams, guiding you toward the life you want to create as you step into your fabulous 50s. Think of it as your very own "dream command center," where every image, word and sparkle (if you're into glitter) holds the power to bring your goals to life. There's real magic in the process of picking out those images and words that make your heart race and your imagination soar. It helps you get crystal clear on what you want, and then it quietly works its magic by embedding those intentions into your subconscious.

Before you know it, you're not just dreaming—you're doing!

Side note: I've got two vision boards hanging up in my bathroom (because, let's face it, the bathroom is a highly frequented spot). One is all about life goals—travel, fitness, that cute little bungalow on the beach—and the other is focused on relationships. Every time I see them during my morning routine, they give me a gentle nudge, reminding me to keep moving forward, even on the days when I just want to hit snooze for the third time.

Here's the best part: making a vision board isn't just about what goes on the board. The real magic happens in the *process*. It's like crafting your personal roadmap to an exciting, joy-filled future, and the journey starts with a little creativity, a stack of magazines and maybe a cup of tea (or a glass of wine—no judgment!).

Materials Needed:

- Poster board or canvas
- Magazines, newspapers, or printed images from the internet
- Scissors
- Glue or double-sided tape
- Markers, colored pencils, or pens
- Stickers, affirmations, or other embellishments (optional)

Step 1: Reflection: Before you go all arts-and-crafts mode, take some time to reflect on what truly matters to you. What are your values, passions and dreams? Think about the areas of your life—relationships, career, health, personal development, hobbies. What experiences do you want to have as you cruise into your 50s and beyond? Take a little time to journal or meditate on this, so you have a clear sense of direction.

Step 2: Gather Materials: Raid your stash of magazines, newspapers or hop online to print out images and words that resonate with your dreams. Keep your eye out for visuals that make you think, *Yes! This is the life I want!* Whether it's a picture of a tropical beach, a quote about resilience or a fancy new hobby, grab it. Your board is all about you!

Step 3: Set the Mood: This part is crucial—set the vibe! Create a space that's inviting, cozy and inspiring. Put on your favorite playlist, light a candle, maybe even put on some comfy slippers. This should feel like a mini-retreat, not a homework assignment. When you're feeling relaxed and inspired, the creative juices will flow!

Step 4: Cut and Collect: Now comes the fun part— grab those scissors and start cutting! Flip through your materials and cut out anything that speaks to you. Don't overthink it—just go with your gut. If a certain image makes you feel excited, snip it out. Trust your instincts here; this is where the magic starts.

Step 5: Organize and Arrange: Now that you've got a pile of inspiring images and words, start laying them out on your board. You can organize them into sections—one for health, one for relationships, one for world domination (kidding... or not)—or just go with the flow and see where things land. The goal is to create a visual that lights you up whenever you look at it.

Step 6: Glue or Tape: When you're happy with the arrangement, it's time to commit. Grab your glue or tape and start sticking everything down. This is when your vision starts to become a tangible reality. There's something satisfying about securing those dreams in place, almost like you're saying, *Yep, this is happening.*

Step 7: Add Personal Touches: Now that the basics are in place, it's time to add some flair! Grab your markers, colored pencils or pens and start adding little personal touches. Write down affirmations, doodle your goals, or add a few quotes that make you feel empowered. If stickers or embellishments make you smile, go ahead and slap them on. Make this board uniquely yours.

Step 8: Reflect on Your Vision: Take a step back and look at your creation. What feelings come up when you look at your board? Does it excite you? Motivate you? Scare you a little in the best possible way? Your vision board should evoke all the emotions that align with the life you're building. Make sure it represents a well-rounded picture of your values and the joy you want to cultivate at this milestone.

Step 9: Display Your Vision Board: Here's the thing about vision boards—they only work if you see them! So, make sure you hang it up in a spot where you'll look at it every day. Whether it's in your bedroom, office, or—like me—in your bathroom, let it be a constant reminder of your goals and dreams. You deserve that daily dose of inspiration!

Step 10: Revisit and Revise: As you move forward, don't be afraid to come back to your board and make adjustments. Your goals will evolve, and so should your vision board. Add new images, change things up, or even start fresh if you feel like it. This isn't a one-time deal—it's a dynamic tool that grows along with you.

Your vision board is more than just a pretty piece of art—it's a visual reminder of the incredible life you're building. It's your personal road map to joy, fulfillment and excitement. So grab your scissors, tap into your creativity and enjoy the process of bringing your future to life, one image at a time. Here's to turning 50 and making it your most inspired year yet!

FIVE

WELLNESS AT 50 AND BEYOND FROM MUSCLES TO MINDSET

"THE PART CAN NEVER BE WELL UNLESS THE WHOLE IS WELL." — PLATO

DURING THE TIME OF WRITING THIS BOOK, I RECEIVED NEWS that a couple of people I know in my age range unexpectedly passed away. I know, here I go again with the morbid mortality talk, but these moments are powerful reminders to lean in closer to our loved ones and take a hard look at our own health.

Wellness at 50 is crucial. It's about finally accepting that your body isn't invincible—it's like a classic car that needs regular maintenance, not just an occasional polish. Plus, staying healthy now means you get to enjoy those senior discounts for many more years to come (I see you, AARP), making you the envy of all your friends still grappling with their 40s.

Wellness is the secret sauce to living your best life, even if that life now involves reading glasses and an odd obsession with comfortable shoes (hallelujah!). It's not just about avoiding doctor visits; it's about ensuring that when you do go, it's for a high-five, not a high blood pressure check. Keeping yourself in good shape means you can keep dancing at weddings, traveling to new places, chasing grandkids, and delivering those legendary "back in my day" stories with plenty of vigor and zest.

While writing this book, I happened to visit my OBGYN for a routine check-up. During the visit, she suggested I undergo genetic testing to see if I was a carrier of any significant disease. I agreed, and a month later, I got the results. It turned out I was at high risk for ovarian and breast cancer. This was a shock, and naturally, I hopped on the internet to consult everyone's favorite doctor—Dr. Google. The most surprising discovery? There are no early screenings for ovarian cancer, which meant I had a big decision to make. The only prevention option for me was surgery, to remove my ovaries and fallopian tubes. That would give me the best fighting chance against the genetic odds I was facing.

In the past, learning I carried that gene would have freaked me out. But now, being armed with knowledge feels empowering, even when the information is scary. Wellness, after all, is about being proactive.

What helps with anything in life? Being as prepared as possible. While there are no guarantees, preparation gives us a fighting chance. In my case, planning for surgery means adopting "pre-op" lifestyle choices that will allow for the best recovery possible. I'm focusing on great nutrition, cutting out inflammatory foods, and keeping my body moving. I'm monitoring my stress levels and choosing a health plan that will keep me out of debt during challenging times. This is how I'm prepping for surgery, and it's a proactive way to live.

And you know what else can help both of us live our healthiest lives now and in the future? Regularly evaluating our wellness. That's where the Wellness Wheel comes in.

What is the Wellness Wheel?

The Wellness Wheel is a model that encompasses various dimensions of well-being, providing a holistic approach to health. In your 50s, addressing each dimension becomes especially important for maintaining overall well-being. If you haven't already visited my website (ontheexhale.com), you can grab the Health and Vitality Inventory to help you dive deeper into each component of wellness.

When it comes to achieving total well-being, a holistic approach that addresses multiple areas of life is key. This includes focusing on **physical, emotional, social, intellectual, occupational, environmental, financial, spiritual, cultural and sleep/rest wellness**. Each of these dimensions plays a vital role in creating a balanced, healthy and fulfilling life. Let's dive deeper into each area and explore practical ways to strengthen them. **You'll score yourself between 1 (not at all) and 10 (mastered) for each, creating awareness of which areas need extra attention.**

Physical Wellness

Physical wellness is about taking care of your body

through regular exercise, proper nutrition and preventative care. Engage in cardiovascular activities like walking, swimming or cycling for heart health. Incorporate strength training and flexibility exercises for overall conditioning. If you're in perimenopause or menopause, talk to your doctor about Hormone Replacement Therapy (HRT), herbal remedies or semiglutides. Men should consider discussing testosterone levels with their doctor. Nutrition is equally important—be sure you're getting enough fiber and protein. Use an online protein calculator to determine how much you should be eating daily to support muscle growth and overall health.

Your Current Score: ___

Emotional Wellness

Emotional wellness means managing stress effectively and nurturing a positive mental state. Stress management techniques like meditation, deep breathing or mindfulness can reduce anxiety and improve mood. Cultivate strong relationships by reaching out to friends or family when you need support. It's important to make time for activities that bring you joy, whether it's painting, gardening or spending time with loved ones. Maintaining emotional wellness is all about consistently doing the things that nourish your soul.

Your Current Score: ___

Social Wellness

Strong social connections are essential for mental and emotional health. Make time to nurture relationships with family and friends, and meet new people who share your interests. Joining a book club or fitness class can be great ways to connect with others. Volunteering or participating in community activities also fosters a sense of purpose and belonging.

Your Current Score: ___

Intellectual Wellness

Challenging your mind keeps it sharp. Read, take up a new hobby or learn something new. Stay curious and open to fresh ideas. Whether it's diving into a good book or tackling a complex puzzle, the goal is to keep your brain engaged and growing.

Your Current Score: ___

Occupational Wellness

Finding purpose and satisfaction in your work is essential. Whether you love your job or are considering a change, maintaining a healthy work-life balance is key. If you're nearing retirement, explore new avenues for fulfillment, like consulting or pursuing hobbies that could become a new occupation.

Your Current Score: ___

Environmental Wellness

Your environment has a significant impact on your well-being. Create a living space that is clean, comfortable and free from clutter. Spending time outdoors or contributing to sustainability efforts can enhance your sense of purpose and well-being.

Your Current Score: ___

Financial Wellness

Financial stability reduces stress and ensures a comfortable future. Evaluate your finances regularly and make plans for retirement. Seeking professional advice can help you manage investments, savings and expenses wisely.

Your Current Score: ___

Spiritual Wellness

Spiritual wellness involves connecting with something greater than yourself, whether through religious practices, meditation or reflection. Engaging in spiritual activities can provide peace, purpose and a sense of connection to the world around you.

Your Current Score: ___

Cultural Wellness

Celebrating your cultural identity can enhance your sense of belonging. Participate in cultural activities, attend festivals or pass down traditions. Appreciating other cultures also broadens your perspectives and enriches your understanding of the world.

Your Current Score: ___

Sleep and Rest

Adequate rest is essential. Prioritize quality sleep by maintaining a consistent routine. Rest is also about recovery—allow your body time to recharge after physical activities to avoid burnout.

Your Current Score: ___

By focusing on these areas, you'll build a well-rounded approach to wellness that supports your mind, body and spirit, allowing you to live your best life with balance and joy.

The Wellness Wheel provides a picture of your current health and wellness. Do you know what else can provide a picture? Your doctor. Here's a list of important health checks and to-dos for turning 50. It's not as fun as a vision board, but its importance is essential to your well-being.

Healthcare at 50: Regular Health Check-ups

- **Annual Physical Exam:** Schedule a comprehensive physical to assess overall health.
- **Blood Pressure Check:** Monitor regularly and have it checked at each visit.
- **Cholesterol Screening:** Discuss cholesterol testing with your provider to assess heart health.
- **Blood Glucose Test:** Screen for diabetes, especially if you have risk factors.
- **Eye Exam:** Get your vision checked and stay on top of potential conditions.

Cancer Screenings:

- **Colorectal Cancer Screening:** Discuss colonoscopy or other tests.
- **Prostate Cancer Screening (Men):** Ask your doctor about PSA tests.
- **Breast Cancer Screening (Women):** Continue regular mammograms.
- **Cervical Cancer Screening (Women):** Keep up with Pap smears and HPV tests.

Bone Health:

- **Bone Density Test:** Talk to your doctor about a test to assess bone health.

Immunizations:

- **Flu Vaccine:** Get it annually.
- **Shingles Vaccine:** Discuss with your provider if appropriate.
- **Pneumococcal Vaccine:** Ensure you're up-to-date.

Lifestyle and Mental Health:

- **Healthy Habits:** Keep up a balanced diet, exercise and sleep.
- **Screening for Depression:** Be open about mental health with your provider.

Dental and Oral Health:

- **Dental Check-up:** Regular cleanings and exams.

Vision and Hearing:

- **Hearing Test:** Consider one if you've noticed changes.

Skin Health:

- **Skin Cancer Check:** Perform regular self-checks and visit a dermatologist.

Lifestyle Reviews:

- **Review Medications:** Go over them with your doctor for possible adjustments.
- **Family Health History:** Update your provider on any changes.

Remember: Take care of your body. It's the only place you have to live!

SIX

KEEP MOVING - WIGGLE IT, JUST A LITTLE BIT

"EXERCISE IS A CELEBRATION OF WHAT YOUR BODY CAN DO, NOT A PUNISHMENT FOR WHAT YOU ATE." — ANONYMOUS

I ONCE WENT TO THIS HARDCORE FITNESS CLASS A FRIEND invited me to. You know, the kind where they yell "burpees!" like it's a term of endearment. My friend, bless his heart, told one of the trainers I was a Zumba instructor, and the trainer lit up. She eagerly shared that her 90-year-old grandmother takes Zumba! 90!! She explained that her grandmother had always been active, and even after a stroke a year and a half ago, she was in such good shape that she bounced right back. Now she's back to doing Zumba and Silver Sneakers workouts. What a woman! Talk about #goals! If there's one takeaway from that story: folks, we've *got* to keep moving. It's the secret sauce!

Recently, at a get-together with some friends, our conversation took a turn, as it does these days:

- "When I stand up, I get so dizzy I feel like I'm going to fall over."
- "I coughed and threw out my back."
- "I slept on my neck wrong four weeks ago, and it *still* doesn't feel right."
- "Is it normal to think it's just a fart, but it turns out to be way more than you bargained for?" (Okay, maybe that last one doesn't quite fit the movement category. But hey, it happens. We're covering all bases here).

Let's face it: as we age, stuff that used to be no big deal starts getting tricky. But the beauty of staying active is that we can change the trajectory of getting older. If you're moving, you're improving!

I've been teaching in the fitness industry for many years, and let me tell you, the happiest people are the ones who move their bodies regularly. And no, they're not all doing Olympic sprints or deadlifting cars. Whether it's Zumba or a nice walk around the neighborhood, it counts! It's all about finding something you enjoy so you can keep at it. Mix up your cardio, strength training, flexibility, and balance exercises for the best results. (And of course, consult your healthcare provider before starting any new program—no wild surprises, please.)

Let's break it down:

Cardio: Whether high or low impact, cardio keeps

your heart happy. Walking is a low-impact option (unless you're speed-walking like you're late for brunch), and cycling or swimming is gentle on your joints. Whatever you choose, your heart will thank you.

Strength Training: In our 50s and beyond, strength training becomes your best friend. It maintains muscle mass, boosts metabolism, and helps prevent falls, osteoporosis, and weight gain. Whether you're squatting with weights or just doing bodyweight exercises like lunges and push-ups, you're keeping yourself strong.

Flexibility: Stretching is the secret to not walking around like a rusty robot (think of the poor Tinman). It keeps your joints mobile, prevents injury, and makes daily life so much easier. Yoga, Pilates, or plain old stretching works wonders. Being able to reach for something without wincing? That's a win.

Balance: Good balance keeps you from becoming besties with the floor. Tai Chi, single-leg stands, or my favorite trick: standing on one foot while brushing your teeth. Two wins in one—minty fresh breath and rock-solid stability!

Most importantly, start slow and keep at it. Consistency is the key. If you're not sure where to begin, working with a fitness professional can be a great way to tailor a routine just for you.

Now, let's get you thinking with this Fitness Interest Survey. It'll help you reflect on what you enjoy, what you want to work on, and where to start. Ready?

Fitness Interest Survey

Welcome to your personalized fitness quiz! No pressure,

just a little insight into how you move (or, you know, don't move) that will help guide us in supporting your wellness journey. Let's dive in—stretch first if you need to.

1. **How would you describe your current experience level with exercise or physical activity?**

   - **Novice:** I have limited experience with exercise or physical activity. (But I have mastered the art of sitting on the couch.)
   - **Intermediate:** I regularly exercise and incorporate a variety of activities. (I've moved beyond beginner, but I still skip leg day sometimes…oops.)
   - **Advanced:** I engage in regular, intense workouts and have extensive experience. (Basically, I'm the human version of a fitness machine.)

1. **What are your primary fitness goals?** (Select all that apply)

   - **Weight Loss:** I want to reduce my body weight. (Not that the scale defines me, but hey, I wouldn't mind making it tremble a little less.)
   - **Muscle Building:** I aim to increase muscle mass and strength. (I'm ready to flex in the mirror and not immediately regret it.)

- **Cardiovascular Health:** I focus on improving heart health and endurance. (I'm tired of pretending I'm looking at my phone while catching my breath.)
- **Flexibility and Mobility:** I want to enhance my range of motion and flexibility. (So I can finally touch my toes without feeling like I'm folding a deck chair.)
- **Stress Reduction:** I use exercise as a way to manage and reduce stress. (Because it's better than stress eating an entire pint of ice cream, right?)
- **General Well-being:** I aim to maintain overall health and well-being. (Translation: I just want to feel good in my own skin.)
- **Other:** Please specify any additional goals you have. (Like becoming a human pretzel? Hey, we won't judge.)

1. **Which types of exercise do you currently enjoy or are interested in trying?** (Select all that apply)

- **Cardio:** Activities like running, cycling, or dancing. (Does running late count as cardio?)
- **Strength Training:** Includes weight lifting, resistance exercises, or bodyweight training. (Lifting groceries counts, right?)

- **Yoga/Pilates:** Focuses on flexibility, balance, and core strength. (Also known as, "Can I do that without falling over?")
- **Group Classes:** Options such as Zumba, spinning, or aerobics. (Perfect if you like sweating with strangers—who doesn't?)
- **Outdoor Activities:** Includes hiking, biking, or walking in nature. (Ah, the great outdoors. As long as there's a bathroom nearby.)
- **Sports:** Participating in sports like tennis, basketball, or soccer. (Or as I like to call it, "an opportunity to trip over my own feet.")
- **Mind-Body Exercises:** Practices like Tai Chi, meditation, or mindful movement. (Because sometimes my mind just needs to catch up with my body.)
- **Other:** Please specify any other types of exercise you are interested in. (Even if it's an Olympic-level walk to the fridge.)

1. **Where do you prefer to exercise?** (Select all that apply)

- **Gym/Fitness Center:** I prefer exercising in a gym or fitness facility. (Where I can pretend I know what all the machines do.)
- **Home:** I prefer working out at home. (Because there's no judgment when I need to pause halfway through to breathe. Or snack.)

- **Outdoors:** I enjoy exercising in outdoor settings like parks or trails. (As long as there's no unexpected wildlife involvement.)
- **Group Classes:** I prefer attending group exercise classes. (Motivation by peer pressure—it works!)
- **Virtual/Online Classes:** I enjoy participating in virtual or online workout sessions. (AKA: Working out in pajamas, and I'm not mad about it.)
- **Other:** Specify any other preferred locations. (Maybe in a parallel universe where I'm a fitness guru.)

1. **How much time can you typically dedicate to exercise per session?**

- **15-30 Minutes:** I usually have about 15-30 minutes per session. (Short, sweet, and sweaty —just the way I like it.)
- **30-45 Minutes:** I can dedicate 30-45 minutes per session. (Long enough to feel accomplished, short enough to avoid total exhaustion.)
- **45-60 Minutes:** I typically exercise for 45-60 minutes per session. (I mean, if I'm already sweaty, I might as well keep going.)
- **60+ Minutes:** I have over an hour to dedicate to exercise per session. (And afterward, I'll need an hour-long nap.)

1. **What time of day do you prefer to exercise?**
   (Select all that apply)

   * **Morning:** I prefer to exercise in the morning.
     (Because the earlier I sweat, the more time I
     have to procrastinate for the rest of the day.)
   * **Afternoon:** I prefer to exercise in the afternoon.
     (Post-lunch, pre-dinner—just trying to make
     my calories count.)
   * **Evening:** I prefer to exercise in the evening.
     (Because there's nothing like a nighttime sweat
     session before collapsing into bed.)
   * **Flexible:** I am flexible and can exercise at
     different times, depending on the day. (Or
     depending on my mood, the weather, or the
     alignment of the planets.)

1. **Are there any specific barriers or challenges
   preventing you from being more active?** (e.g.,
   time constraints, health concerns, lack of
   motivation, Netflix binges, a deep emotional
   attachment to your couch, etc.)

Reflecting on Your Responses

Take a deep breath (optional) and look over your
answers. Let's break it down:

   * **Experience Level:** If you're a novice, no
     worries! Start slow, and don't compare yourself
     to that one friend who runs marathons before

breakfast. For intermediate or advanced movers, maybe it's time to spice up your routine—have you tried something wild like goat yoga?

- **Fitness Goals:** What's driving you? Whether it's sculpting those muscles or simply fitting into your favorite jeans, your goals give you direction. And if that direction includes chocolate breaks… we won't tell.
- **Exercise Preferences:** If you love an activity, make it a regular thing! Hate it? Let it go faster than a bad first date.
- **Exercise Environment:** You're not alone if your living room has doubled as your gym. But if you're craving fresh air, maybe it's time to venture outside. Who knows, maybe the squirrels will cheer you on.
- **Time Commitment:** No need to stress about cramming a 2-hour workout into your day. Just do what you can—whether it's a solid 15 minutes or a full hour. Every little bit counts!
- **Preferred Exercise Time:** Morning bird? Night owl? Or do you just workout when the spirit moves you? Whatever your answer, find what works best for you—and stick with it.
- **Barriers to Physical Activity:** We all have them. Whether it's Netflix's latest hit series or the gravitational pull of your couch, the trick is to recognize those obstacles and start with small steps to overcome them. Just don't trip over

those steps—unless it's part of your new balance routine!

So, what's the takeaway here? Keep moving. Whatever it is—whether it's trying out the *number one* sport in America (hello, Pickleball!) or dancing around your living room—it's all good. If you're stuck, use this quiz to guide you toward movement you enjoy and can stick with. Remember—people who move their bodies are happier. And who doesn't want an extra slice of happy?

SEVEN
YOUR GOLDEN COMMUNITY - LESS DRAMA, MORE KARMA

"FRIENDSHIP IS BORN AT THAT MOMENT WHEN ONE PERSON SAYS TO ANOTHER, 'WHAT! YOU TOO? I THOUGHT I WAS THE ONLY ONE.'" – C.S. LEWIS

HITTING THE BIG 5-0 OFTEN COMES WITH A REALIZATION: meaningful relationships are like fine wine—they only get better with time, provided you handle them with care. At this stage of life, our connections might have shifted, evolved or even taken a sabbatical, but the beauty of it all is that we have the chance to reignite, renew, release or deepen these bonds. Setting the intention to nurture and cherish our relationships isn't just a good idea; it's a recipe for a happier, richer life. Let's dive in now and fine-tune our current and future connections. After all, it takes a village, and we want to make sure ours is thriving.

Let's take a moment to play relationship detective. Pull out your imaginary magnifying glass and reflect on your connections—family, friends, colleagues. Think back to *Chapter 2: The Great Release,* where we discussed reason, season and lifetime relationships. Which ones still give you those warm fuzzies, and which ones feel more like a chilly breeze? You may be thinking, *Why do I have to keep examining relationships?* Well, as I told my kids during their growing-up years, "You are the five people you choose to spend the most time with." Identifying relationships that are thriving, and those that might need a little TLC, is key. Tools for evaluating these connections can be as simple as asking yourself: *"Do I feel energized and appreciated after spending time with this person, or do I need a nap and a glass of wine?"* Remember, relationships are meant to lift you up, not drag you down.

Strengthening connections often starts with the power of active listening. Picture this: you're having a conversation, and instead of planning your grocery list in your head, you're actually engaged. Empathy is key here. Try to see things from the other person's perspective. If they're talking about their latest hobby, put yourself in their shoes—even if it's a hobby you wouldn't touch with a 10-foot pole. Quality time is also essential. It's not about cramming in as many hangouts as possible; it's about making those moments together count, even if it's just a shared chuckle over a cup of coffee.

Let's face it, building new friendships at 50 can feel a bit like dating all over again. It's nerve-wracking but also exciting. Go to places where your ideal community can be found. Do you want be around people who are into mindfulness? Consider yoga or retreats. Want to be around a fun, healthy, and active crowd? Try team sports like pickleball. Dive into community activities, clubs, or classes where people gather around shared interests. Who knows? You might just find your new best friend in a pottery class or a music group. Mentorship is another great way to forge new connections. Be open to learning from others, and don't shy away from sharing your own experiences. After all, wisdom is meant to be passed around like a good piece of chocolate.

Now, sometimes, relationships can feel like a roller coaster with a few too many loops. Managing challenging relationships requires finesse. Start with honesty and tact —address issues openly, but remember, you're aiming for a solution, not a showdown. Setting boundaries is crucial. Think of them as your personal "do not disturb" sign. It's OK to step back from relationships that constantly leave you feeling like you've been hit by a tidal wave of negativity. Letting go can be tough, but sometimes it's the healthiest choice for both parties. Surround yourself with people who help bring out one of the best sides of yourself and return the favor.

If you are currently in partnership (or marriage with someone), what are ways that you both can refresh your relationship? We change as life changes. If you are empty nesters, it might be time to get to know each other again and who you are when parenting isn't the main focus. Be open to talking about what is exciting and what is scary for this new stage of life and find out how to support and love your partner best. Get curious.

Let's talk about relationships and technology—the

double-edged sword of modern life. On one hand, it keeps us connected with loved ones no matter where they are. On the other hand, it sometimes feels like we're talking to screens more than to real people. Embrace technology as a tool to keep those bonds alive, but don't let it replace face-to-face interactions. Video calls are great, but there's nothing quite like a good old-fashioned hug—or at least a warm handshake. Explore new apps and platforms to stay in touch, but make sure they complement, not replace, real-world interactions. Balance is key, like finding the perfect amount of cream in your coffee.

On that same note, what is your relationship feeling like with technology? Do you feel like you are always connected (guilty!)? Do you feel like you are jonesing for your phone when you are away from it? Consider where this relationship is in your life and where it falls under your priorities and values. (Check out *Experience #26* of when I did a 24-hour phone fast). Recently, someone said to me, "We are more 'tech-connected' than ever, but we are starved for connection." It resonated deeply because, as humans, we need real, tangible connections. It's a basic need, and it's perfectly OK to acknowledge that and to find the balance.

Real-life interactions are exactly what they say: REAL. Take my close girlfriends from high school, for example. Every two years, we go on a girls' trip, even though we are scattered across the country. It takes time, planning, and a bit of money, but every time we get together, my cup runneth over. We reminisce about our younger years, share what's happening in our current lives, and create new memories. I also have other close girlfriends, like two women I met at a previous job where we bonded over our work as health coaches. Though we live in different places, we share the same energy, and when we talk or get together, it's pure magic (and lots of woo).

Even locally, I've formed a group of close friends through teaching Zumba—people who add to my life in a healthy atmosphere. And believe it or not, I've even transitioned a few dating-app matches into genuine friendships. One friend I met over 20 years ago when we were both ESL teachers has become a lifelong confidant. These examples are part of what I call my "Golden Community." Your own Golden Community doesn't have to come from just one place—it's about who adds value to your life.

Strong relationships are like daily doses of happiness vitamins. They can boost your mood, reduce stress and make life's challenges a bit easier to handle. Think of your relationships as your personal cheer squad—they're there to lift you up, support you, and make you laugh until you cry. On the flip side, relationships that drain your energy can be more detrimental than that last slice of cake you didn't really need. Recognizing and nurturing the positive connections in your life can enhance your overall well-being, turning everyday moments into sources of joy.

Cultivating relationships is an ongoing adventure, not a one-time project. By reflecting on your current connections, strengthening existing bonds, and welcoming new ones, you're crafting a network that supports and enriches your life. Remember, relationships are like gardening—tend to them with love and patience, and they'll bloom beautifully. So, keep nurturing those connections, stay proactive, and enjoy the wonderful impact that meaningful relationships bring to your life.

Connections Activity

Identify Your Core Connections: Write down 3-5 people who are very important to you. These are individuals who significantly impact your life, whether through friendship, family ties, or meaningful

Person #1:

Person #2:

Person #3:

Person #4:

Person #5:

- Reflect on Strengthening Your Bonds: Consider the following ways to enhance and deepen these relationships:
- **Regular Communication:** Make an effort to reach out frequently, whether through phone calls, texts or in-person meetings.
- **Quality Time:** Spend meaningful time together, engaging in activities that you both enjoy and that strengthen your connection.
- **Express Appreciation:** Regularly express gratitude and appreciation for their presence and support in your life.

- **Offer Support:** Be there for them in times of need, offering help, advice, or simply a listening ear.
- **Goals:** Find common interests or goals that you can pursue together, fostering a stronger sense of partnership.

Evaluate Your Relationships: Are there other individuals you would like to include or exclude from this list? Reflect on your current relationships and consider if there are people who you would like to strengthen connections with or possibly distance yourself from.

- **New Additions:** Are there individuals who have recently become important or who you would like to get to know better?
- **Re-evaluation:** Are there relationships that no longer align with your values or that may be draining your energy? Consider if adjustments are needed to maintain a healthy and positive community.

By actively engaging in these practices, you can expand your network, deepen existing relationships, and foster a supportive and enriching community around you.

EIGHT
AUTHENTICITY AND THE REAL YOU - TAKING OFF THE MASK

"AUTHENTICITY IS THE DAILY PRACTICE OF LETTING GO OF WHO WE THINK WE'RE SUPPOSED TO BE AND EMBRACING WHO WE ARE." — BRENÉ BROWN

IN A WORLD THAT OFTEN ENCOURAGES US TO WEAR MASKS—whether for social acceptance, career success, or to avoid the dreaded "What were you thinking?" looks from family—authenticity can seem elusive. Yet, as I approached 50, I realized that living an authentic life is not just a choice; it's a necessity for true happiness. Otherwise, I'd end up a 70-year-old with a closet full of masks and no real clue who I actually was underneath. This chapter is about embracing the power of authenticity, shedding those layers of pretense, and stepping into who *you* are—unapologetically and, yes, a little awkwardly at times. You've already done the pre-work by examining your past, values and strengths. Now,

71

let's dive into making sure you know who you are at the core.

Let's be honest: the journey to authenticity doesn't happen overnight. It's a bit like untangling the Christmas lights you tossed in a box back in January—you'll need some time, patience, and maybe a little help from a friend who can see things more clearly than you. Early on in life, we're often too busy trying to blend in, please others and fit into the strange boxes society hands us. People-pleasers, I see you (and me!). By the time we're 50, though, we've lived enough to realize that most of those boxes aren't even the right size.

Authenticity isn't about getting it all right—it's about being real. It's about showing up as yourself, flaws and all, even if that means admitting you don't know what you're doing half the time. (Pro tip: Most people don't.)

By the time you hit 50, something magical happens: you realize you really don't care what most people think anymore. Seriously, it's like a superpower. All those masks you wore in your 20s and 30s—the "perfect" professional, the "always strong" friend, the "I totally have my life together" person? Yeah, they start to feel a little itchy like an uncomfortable scratchy garment. So, off they come.

For me, this started showing up in dating. In my late 30s, after my divorce, I went on many dates. I took pride in the fact that nearly every guy asked for a second date. I thought, *Look at me. Everyone wants a second date. I am accepted and valued, cherished and adored.* Except... I wasn't. I was showing up to these dates as I thought they would want me to be and making it all about the other person. While it's important to give space for your dates to share about themselves, I made them the star and gave them all my energy! Naturally, they wanted a second date because it was all about them. When I got closer to 50, that changed. I only wanted to be in a relationship with someone who could provide equal space for me as I was providing for them. I was tired, y'all. Guess what happened? Fewer dates. Fewer second dates. But a much more real me.

We tend to think of authenticity as strength, but let's not sugarcoat it—authenticity is messy. It's about being vulnerable, which, let's face it, is like walking around in your pajamas inside out in public: not exactly comfortable, but it shows people who you really are.

When I started being honest about my struggles— whether with aging, relationships or that weird crick in my back from sleeping wrong—something surprising happened: people connected with me more deeply. Turns out, everyone's walking around with their own secret cricks, too. Authenticity breeds connection, and connection is what makes life rich.

Vulnerability doesn't make you weak; it makes you real. Plus, let's be honest: nobody likes a person who pretends to have it all figured out. (That person is probably losing their mind in private.) So, when I let go of pretending to be "strong" all the time, I found strength in being myself.

Living authentically isn't a one-time decision—it's like working out: you've got to do it regularly, or your "authenticity muscles" get flabby. So, here's what that looks like for me on a daily basis:

- **Listening to My Gut**: And no, I don't mean the extra slice of pizza. I mean trusting my instincts, even when they go against logic. If something feels off, I don't need to rationalize it. I just go with it—like walking away from relationships or situations that didn't feel right.
- **Speaking My Truth**: Honestly, sometimes this is the hardest. It means being brave enough to say things like, "Actually, I don't like pineapple on pizza," even if it means losing friends. Authenticity isn't for the faint of heart.
- **Setting Boundaries**: I've mastered the art of saying "No," and it's been life-changing. (No, really. Try it.) If something doesn't align with my values or energy, I pass. No guilt, no drama —just a peaceful night at home with my dogs.
- **Accepting Imperfection**: This is a big one. Perfection? Overrated. Flaws? They're interesting. Plus, imperfection gives us all something to laugh about, and I've found humor to be the ultimate antidote to taking myself too seriously.

There's an amazing freedom that comes with living authentically. It's like taking off a pair of shoes that are two sizes too small—you can finally breathe. When you're not trying to be someone else, you get to focus on

74

just being you. And here's the best part: when you embrace your quirks, your flaws, your weird sense of humor, and all the things that make you unique, people are drawn to you. Not to the version of you they think they want, but to you.

So, as you reflect on your own life, ask yourself: Where am I not being authentic? What masks am I still holding onto? And maybe most importantly: Do I like pineapple on pizza? Because that's really what it's all about—being real with yourself in the big stuff and the little stuff (not so much about the pineapple). Authenticity may not always be easy, but I promise you this: it's a whole lot more fun.

NINE
YOUR LEGACY - LEAVING FOOTPRINTS WITHOUT CRUSHING THE GRASS

"CARVE YOUR NAME ON HEARTS, NOT TOMBSTONES." — SHANNON L. ALDER

ONE LOS ANGELES SUMMER NIGHT IN AUGUST OF 2024, MY cousin Amy, her husband Rob, and their two teenage boys were eating dinner at home. Rob went to go to the bathroom and never came back. At age 52, his death shocked us all and my cousin Amy, her boys, and the rest of the family were left sorting through the grief. I flew out from Texas for the funeral and my dad, sister and her family drove from Arizona.

The day of the funeral, we went to Hillside Memorial Park in Los Angeles. The instructions were to wear Hawaiian clothes since Rob loved Hawaii and Jimmy Buffet. When we pulled into Hillside and told the gate guard the funeral we were attending, he said, "There are so many people here for this service today. He must have been very loved." Hundreds of people were in attendance with bright colored shirts.

The words of the gate guard kept coming back to me. "He must have been very loved." Whether it is with hundreds of people or just a few, the life we live has an effect on others. We all eventually meet our end. We are our legacy. Let's make it a good one.

Planning your legacy might sound a bit like writing a grand farewell letter to the world—but don't worry, we're going to make it as enjoyable as possible! While leaving behind a meaningful impact is serious business, there's no reason we can't have a little fun while doing it. So, grab a cup of water, coffee, or something stronger, and let's dive into planning your legendary exit with a smile.

Define Your Core Values and Beliefs:

Think about the values that have shaped your life (think back to Chapter 3) —these will be your guiding light when it comes to your legacy. And hey, if "eating pizza on Fridays" makes the list, own it!

What principles have guided your life decisions (even the questionable ones)?

Which values do you want to leave behind (besides the secret family recipe for perfect lasagna)?

Examples of core values: kindness, loyalty, always returning library books on time, never skipping dessert.

Action Step:

Write a personal mission statement that sums up what you stand for—just remember to keep it under 10 pages.

Identify Your Impact on Others:

Take a moment to reflect on how you've left your mark on this world. Maybe you've been a mentor, a friend, or the person everyone calls when they can't figure out how to change their Wi-Fi password.

How have you made people's lives better (or at least a little more fun)?

Which causes, communities, or Netflix shows have been important to you?

What legacy do you want to leave (besides that hilarious story about the time you accidentally texted your boss instead of your friend)?

Action Step:

Pinpoint three projects or actions that reflect your values and make sure your legacy is more than just a collection of funny anecdotes (although, let's be honest, those are gold).

Capture Your Life Lessons:

We all know life is full of lessons, many of them learned the hard way—like the time you realized putting foil in the microwave was a bad idea. What nuggets of wisdom do you want to pass on?

What life lessons are too important to forget (like how to make a proper cup of coffee)?

Are there stories or experiences you want to share, like that one time in college that's still technically classified?

Action Step:

Write letters or record videos for your loved ones. This is your chance to pass down both wisdom *and* embarrassing stories for future generations.

Plan Your Personal Legacy Projects:

Your legacy can go beyond memories. Maybe you have unfinished creative projects or simply want to ensure your dog Fluffy is remembered as the true hero they were.

Got any creative works, unfinished business, or dreams of being remembered as a local legend?

How can you ensure these projects keep going, even if your DIY scrapbook isn't done yet?

Action Step:

Set up a plan for your projects to carry on without you. Whether it's a novel, a foundation, or just making sure the world's supply of cat memes continues—leave your mark!

Consider Your Relationships and Emotional Legacy:

Let's get real for a second. The connections we build throughout our lives are what people will truly remember —whether it's for your endless kindness, or your unrivaled ability to dominate at family board games.

How do you want to be remembered in your relationships (as the one who always made everyone laugh or as the designated holiday meal chef)?

Got any apologies, thanks or shout-outs to give while you're still around?

Action Step:

Strengthen those important relationships. Mend fences, say thank you, and if you're holding a grudge about that Monopoly game from 2010—let it go. Your legacy will thank you.

Reflect on How You Want Your Funeral to Be:

Ah yes, the grand finale. Planning your funeral doesn't have to be morbid—it can be a reflection of your life, your personality, and maybe even your sense of humor.

Do you want a serious ceremony or more of a "let's celebrate with cake and stories" vibe?

. . .

Any songs, readings, or dad jokes you want thrown in?

Who gets to speak at your funeral, and should you give them a time limit to avoid rambling?

Funeral Planning Considerations:

- **Type of ceremony**: Traditional, outdoor gathering, or a "watch my life highlight reel while eating tacos" event.
- **Location**: Church, backyard, favorite beach or that restaurant where everyone knows your name.
- **Music and readings**: Go for something meaningful, but if "Don't Stop Believin'" is your jam, by all means, play it!
- **Personal touches**: Want your guests to wear Hawaiian shirts or release biodegradable balloons? Make it happen!
- **Burial or cremation preferences**: Whether it's traditional burial or having your ashes shot out of a cannon—just be clear.

Action Step:

Write down your funeral preferences and share them with loved ones (maybe over dinner, for fun).

. . .

Create a Will and Estate Plan:

Let's get practical for a second—who's going to get that cherished Star Wars action figure collection? Estate planning ensures that your assets go to the right people (and that no one fights over your vintage record player).

Do you have a will in place? If not, consider making one before that "someday" turns into "today."

Who will be your beneficiaries, and have you left anything to charity (or your pets)?

Should you set up a trust, or at least a fund to cover someone else's future pizza deliveries?

<u>**Action Step:**</u>

Work with a professional to set up your estate plan. You want to make sure your prized possessions (and quirky mementos) are in good hands.

Leave a Digital Legacy:

In the digital age, your online presence is a big part of your legacy. What will happen to your social media accounts, blogs, or that YouTube channel where you posted your cooking fails?

How do you want your digital legacy handled (including all those early selfies from 2012)?

. . .

Do you want a farewell post on Instagram, or a special playlist dedicated to you on Spotify?

Action Step:

Use digital estate planning tools to ensure your digital afterlife is as curated as you want it to be.

Write Your Own Obituary:

Don't wait for someone else to write your life story—this is your chance to tell it like it is! Who knows your quirks, accomplishments, and that "one time in Vegas" better than you?

- How would you describe the highs, lows and hilarious in-betweens of your life?

- What achievements or random life events do you want to highlight (like winning that pie-eating contest)?

Action Step:

Draft your own obituary, whether it's funny, poignant, or just an excuse to finally get the last word.

. . .

Create and Ongoing Legacy of Kindness and Giving:

Why not leave a legacy of kindness that lives on long after you do? Whether it's setting up a scholarship, starting a charitable foundation, or just making sure someone keeps your secret stash of chocolate well-stocked.

- How can you keep spreading kindness, even after you're gone?

- What causes do you care about, and how can future generations carry on your legacy of giving (or cookie-baking)?

Action Step:

If you are feeling inspired to do so, set up a charitable fund or legacy project that will keep your name (and your kindness) alive.

Planning your legacy doesn't have to be all somber—it's an opportunity to reflect on your life, your quirks, and how you want to be remembered. So, go ahead and tackle this with a blend of thoughtfulness and humor. After all, it's your story—make it a good one!

TEN

YOUR TURN - PLANNING YOUR "HELL YES" EXPERIENCES

"LIFE IS EITHER A DARING ADVENTURE OR NOTHING AT ALL." – HELEN KELLER

WHEN WE STOP TRYING NEW THINGS, OUR BRAINS CAN GET too comfortable and start to slow down. Think of your brain as a muscle—it thrives on a good workout. Without fresh challenges, it becomes lazy. Your memory might not stay as sharp, decision-making and problem-solving could feel tougher, and life can start to feel monotonous. Without the dopamine hit that comes from new experiences, you might even find yourself less motivated and a bit down. The real kicker? The more we avoid trying new things, the more our brain's "fear center" kicks in, making change seem scarier than it really is.

Take a moment and think back to a time you tried something new. Maybe it was a recipe, a sport, a new social situation, a job, or learning a computer program. What was the experience like?

When we try something new, our brain creates pathways that strengthen with repetition, making the task easier over time. Think of learning to play the guitar—at first, it feels awkward to find the right strings, but with practice, those neural connections strengthen, and soon it becomes second nature. This process is supported by dopamine, the neurotransmitter linked to pleasure and reward. When we engage in new activities, dopamine is released, motivating us to repeat the behavior. For example, after successfully rock climbing for the first time, the dopamine rush leaves you feeling proud and eager to try again.

Several other parts of the brain work together when we take on something unfamiliar. The amygdala, responsible for processing emotions like fear and excitement, becomes highly active, making the experience more memorable—like the nervous energy you feel when giving a public speech. The hippocampus, essential for memory formation, helps encode these new experiences into long-term memory. When you explore a new city without a map, your hippocampus helps you store those routes, making the unfamiliar territory more recognizable over time. Lastly, the frontal lobe, which manages decision-making and problem-solving, kicks in as you navigate these new tasks. Whether you're cooking a new recipe or learning a new skill, your brain is actively working to adapt. No one wants a mushy brain and keeping it sharp takes effort. Ready to start planning experiences that will keep your brain engaged and your life fulfilling? It's time!

I'm about to say something, and it may take a moment to sink in. Ready? Take a big breath. Here it goes: **We are responsible for how we feel.** Not our boss. Not our kids. Not our partner. Dang it! It's so much easier to blame someone else, isn't it? But nope, we're the ones on the hook for how we feel in any situation.

Now, let's translate that to experiences. You could be sitting in your living room or standing on top of the tallest mountain with stunning views, and you could feel joy in both places. Or, you could feel miserable. The choice is yours. That means if you choose an experience you think will rock your world, remember: the real rocking happens on the inside. You set the stage, and you set the mood.

Does that feel daunting? Maybe a little. But it's also freeing to know that you get to create your own feelings, and everyone else gets to create theirs! Knowing this as you head into your planning session is important because you get to decide who (if anyone) joins you and how you feel along the way.

Ready? This is your DIY Planning Session for **Things to Try at 50 (or any age!)**. I created this guide to help you plan a list of exciting and fulfilling activities as you enter this new chapter of your life. Think of it as a blueprint or roadmap for adding spice and fun to your days.

But first, let me say this: **This is NOT a to-do list.** This is a **DREAMY, DELICIOUS, FUN, ADVENTUROUS, HELL YES LIST.** My suggestion? Make sure you're in the right mindset when going through this guide. Take deep breaths. Pray or meditate beforehand. Maybe go for a walk to clear your head and spark ideas. This shouldn't feel like "one more thing you have to do." If you're stressed, overwhelmed, tired, or sad, it's harder to tap into what truly lights you up.

Your Planning Guide

How to Use this Guide: Go through each category. If something feels like a *HELL YES* for you, circle it. If it's a maybe, put a ? by it. If it's a *hell no*, cross it out.

Remember—this is your list and your life! There are no right or wrong answers, just your own authentic heart and soul guiding you. Now, go have some fun!

Reflect on Future Achievements and Aspirations:

- What I hope to still achieve/do in this life:

Health and Wellness:

Prioritize your well-being by incorporating health-focused activities into your plan.

- Explore a new fitness routine or sport. Is there a sport or routine you have been wanting to try?
- Try meditation or yoga for mental and physical well-being.
- Schedule regular health check-ups and screenings (check back to the chapter on the Wellness Wheel that gives a list of check-ups and screenings.)

- Experiment with different wellness practices like tai chi, Pilates, or martial arts.
- Take on a physical challenge like a marathon, triathlon or a long-distance bike ride.
- Explore holistic health approaches like acupuncture, aromatherapy or massage therapy.
- Other:

Travel and Adventure:

Feed your sense of adventure by planning exciting travel experiences.

- Create a bucket list of destinations you've always wanted to visit.
- Consider a solo trip for self-discovery.
- Explore your local area and discover hidden gems.
- Plan a road trip with no set itinerary, allowing spontaneous adventures.
- Try "voluntourism" and combine travel with volunteering for a cause you're passionate about.
- Take a nature-based trip like camping, hiking in national parks or visiting remote islands.
- Other:

Learn Something New:

Stimulate your mind by taking up new hobbies or learning new skills.

- Enroll in a class or workshop that interests you.
- Learn to play a musical instrument or speak a new language.
- Dive into literature or explore art and culture.
- Take up a DIY project like woodworking, knitting or gardening.
- Join a book club, discussion group, or start a blog on a topic you love.
- Explore online courses on subjects ranging from history to coding to astronomy.
- Other:

Connect with Loved Ones:

Strengthen relationships with family and friends.

- Plan a memorable celebration with loved ones.
- Schedule regular gatherings or trips with friends and family.
- Consider volunteering together for a meaningful experience.
- Start a tradition like a monthly game night, movie marathon or themed dinner party.
- Organize a family reunion or a big group trip.

- Create a shared hobby or project, like a family scrapbook or a community garden.
- Other:

Culinary Adventures:

Explore your culinary creativity and expand your palate.

- Take a cooking class or experiment with new recipes.
- Try dining at unique or exotic restaurants.
- Host a themed dinner party for friends and family.
- Go to a Michelin Star or James Beard award-winning restaurant.
- Explore food tours or cooking vacations in different regions or countries.
- Start a food blog or Instagram page to document your culinary journey.
- Experiment with dietary changes, like going vegan for a month or trying out intermittent fasting.
- Other:

Personal Growth and Development:

Invest in your personal growth and self-discovery.

- Set personal development goals for the next decade.
- Consider therapy or coaching for personal insights.
- Engage in activities that boost confidence and self-esteem.
- Create a vision board to visualize your goals and dreams for the future.
- Attend a personal growth retreat or seminar focused on mindfulness, leadership or spirituality.
- Start journaling regularly to reflect on your thoughts, emotions and progress.
- Other:

Creative Pursuits

Unleash your creativity through various artistic outlets.

- Take up painting, photography or writing.
- Attend art shows, concerts or theater performances.
- Express yourself through creative projects.
- Join a creative community or club to share ideas and inspiration.
- Experiment with different forms of art like pottery, sculpture or digital design.

- Create the song that has been forming in your heart and mind, and get it on paper.
- Start a long-term creative project, like writing a novel, creating a photo series or making a short film.
- Other:

Adventure Sports

Push your limits and try thrilling adventure sports.

- Consider activities like skydiving, rock climbing or zip-lining.
- Join a sports club or group for camaraderie and fun.
- Embrace the adrenaline rush and conquer fears.
- Try water sports like surfing, scuba diving or white-water rafting.
- Explore winter sports like skiing, snowboarding or ice climbing.
- Take up an endurance sport, such as marathon running, cycling or triathlons.
- Other:

Spirituality

Explore new dimensions of your spiritual journey and growth.

- Try practices like meditation, yoga or breathwork.
- Attend a spiritual retreat or silent meditation retreat.
- Participate in a sound bath or crystal healing session.
- Experience energy work such as Reiki, acupuncture or chakra balancing.
- Join a spiritual or metaphysical group for community and support.
- Explore practices like tarot, astrology or numerology for self-awareness.
- Attend a holistic fair or spiritual workshop.
- Get involved in your faith group by attending regular services or participating in study groups.
- Volunteer with a religious organization or charity for a deeper connection to your faith.
- Other:

Gratitude and Mindfulness

Cultivate gratitude and mindfulness for a more fulfilling life.

- Keep a gratitude journal to focus on positive aspects.
- Practice mindfulness through meditation or nature walks.

- Appreciate the present moment and savor life's experiences.
- Start a daily or weekly meditation practice, using apps or guided sessions.
- Engage in mindful movement practices like yoga, tai chi or walking meditation.
- Create a space in your home dedicated to mindfulness and relaxation, filled with items that bring you peace.
- Other:

Are there ideas you have that weren't mentioned above? Use this area to write them down:

OK, how did that feel? Did that get your excitement juices flowing? Now it is time to write down your top experience *Hell Yes* experiences. If you feel like you can only come up with one or two, that's great! Embrace and focus on those. If you have 4,123 ideas, then that is great too. This is your brainstorming session. There are no limits or rules.

1.
2.
3.
4.
5.
6.

7.

8.

9.

10.

But wait...you don't want to just write them down and tuck them away on Fantasy Island. Let's get some time frames and/or dates on the calendar.

Action Step:

Go back to that list of your top 10 and write WHEN you want to start it by. If it feels too big to start the entire experience, what is one first step you can take towards that experience? For example, if you want to go on a cruise to the Bahamas, but planning an entire trip overwhelms you, a first step could look like contacting a travel agent or seeing what cruise ships sail to the Bahamas. If writing a book is on your list (speaking from experience), commit to writing one page a day or one chapter a week. If it feels like "work" then does it belong on your top five list?

My list:

Experience #1:

First Step:

Experience #2:

First Step:

Experience #3:

First Step:

Experience #4:

First Step:

Experience #5:

First Step:

Experience #6:

First Step:

Experience #7:

First Step:

Experience #8:

First Step:

Experience #9:

First Step:

Experience #10:

First Step:

Look at you! Making plans and putting your zest into overdrive. If you are still stuck, jump ahead to the next chapters of the 50 things I did to give you some ideas. Revisit this often. Change it whenever. These are your dreams! Reserve the right to stay flexible and change them as needed. Go shine, you gorgeous human! This isn't a dress rehearsal. You are the star of your life.

PART ONE
50 NEW EXPERIENCES

YOU DID WHAT?

As you navigated your way through your past and set forth on how you want to live now and, in the future, are you feeling excited? Nervous? Scared as hell? I can relate.

When I thought about turning 50, I knew it couldn't just be a year, or another birthday, or a number. It had to be celebrated by doing something special. What could I do to commemorate this? Throw a big party? Take a big trip? Get my first tattoo? I had already visited all 50 states. I had done a lot of solo travel both domestically and internationally. I have tried many new things. What could I do to really celebrate this entire year?

One day, while thinking about ways to really bring in this epic number, it came to me. I could *intentionally* try 50 new experiences I have never tried before during the entire year I turned 50 (2024). Now, I am not someone who has ever shied away from new experiences. I have a whole list of unique happenings that I have done in my life. But to intentionally do 50 new things in one year, now that was something.

I started my 50 adventures in January 2024 and finished my last experience at the end of October. Some of the experiences were always on my bucket list (like riding in a hot air balloon). Others I found along the way through my own searching online (like on Facebook Events, Eventbrite or word of mouth). Sometimes, the experience came to me without planning. I found myself open to listening to new experiences with even more attuned listening and being open. And because of that, I tried things that never crossed my mind (like fencing and attending a séance).

Some of the experiences were big, and some weren't. But they expanded me in one way or another. I delved into the fact that they didn't have to be huge and life-changing to be a new experience. After all, life is made of the big and small, and so were the experiences. Some were corny and humorous. Others life-changing and thought-provoking. Some just plain fun! Each one is now a memory of my 50th year, a treasure for sure. I hope that they inspire you and give you both ideas and drive to create your own beautiful year. Most importantly, these experiences show something I appreciate most of all. I lived, and I hope they inspire you too as well.

EXPERIENCE #1: TAKE MY GRANDDAUGHTER ON AN EPIC TRIP

In January of this year, I decided to do something a little out of the ordinary—I booked airline tickets to Arizona to surprise my dad for the day. But I wasn't going alone; I was bringing along my 4 ½-year-old granddaughter, Grace. The whole idea was to make it a fun, memorable adventure for both of us, and surprise my dad in the process. On Christmas morning, I was delighted to share the news with Grace through a scavenger hunt that I had meticulously planned out. I was expecting wide-eyed excitement and maybe a little jumping up and down. Instead, when she finally pieced together the big reveal, she looked up at me and said, "Are we leaving now?" When I told her we weren't leaving immediately, she lost interest faster than you can say "new toys," and went back to playing with her other Christmas presents. Kids these days! (I guess that's the official phrase that marks my transition into grumpy old person status.)

Flying with kids is always an adventure—and I mean

that in the most unpredictable, hold-on-to-your-sanity kind of way. The last time Grace was on a plane, she was just an infant, and her mom was there to help wrangle her. This time, it was going to be just the two of us, so I knew I needed to prepare her (and myself) for the journey. In our dining room, I set up three chairs in a row to mimic airplane seats, and we practiced sitting down, putting on our imaginary seatbelts, and pretending to look out the imaginary window at the tiny cars and buildings below. I even put on my best "flight attendant" voice to explain that she'd have to carry her own backpack. If you're laughing right now, you've got the right idea—because let's be real, that didn't happen. I ended up being the pack mule, as expected.

The actual day of our flight started early—so early, in fact, that even the sun wasn't ready to greet us. As we drove to the airport, Grace was fascinated by the tall buildings she had never seen before, which she quickly dubbed "castles." I guess Corporate America has a certain fairytale charm when you're 4 ½ years old.

We made it to the airport, breezed through security, and spent some time admiring the planes out the windows. Grace was absolutely mesmerized by the idea that these giant metal birds could actually fly. Our flight was completely full, so Grace got the coveted window seat, I was in the middle, and a pilot—who wasn't flying our plane, —was in the aisle seat. As we took off, Grace was glued to the window, exclaiming how tiny everything looked. When we reached the clouds, she excitedly pointed out how they looked like waffles. I have to admit, she was onto something there. Or maybe I was just hungry. The window-gazing lasted a solid 10 minutes before the novelty wore off and she turned her attention to more pressing matters: snacks and her tablet. Before I knew it, she had conked out on my lap for the rest of the flight.

Upon landing, we were greeted by my sister, three teenage nephews, and my brother-in-law. Grace immediately bonded with her cousins, who she referred to simply as "cousins" for the rest of the trip. No names necessary, just a collective noun that fit the bill. Our first mission was to surprise my dad at brunch. He knew I was coming, but had no idea that Grace was with me. When she jumped out and yelled "Surprise!" his face was priceless. Grace melted into his arms, and it was clear that this surprise was a huge success.

After gobbling down brunch (because who can resist good food when you're in great company?), we headed to the Phoenix Children's Museum. Now, let me just say, this museum is the kind that makes you reconsider your stance on museums altogether. Forget the stuffy art museums of my childhood that had me stifling yawns and daydreaming about escape routes—this place was filled with interactive fun! There was an art-inspired, enormous jungle gym, tunnels, a human car (bike) wash, and rooms full of arts and crafts. The museum even had noodles—the kind you use in swimming pools—that kids could run through. Grace was in her element, and honestly, so was I. After playing there for a couple of hours the museum was about to close, and we were about to head to a nice meal, when I got some new information on the flight.

Our flight home got bumped to an earlier time, so our family dinner plans shifted to dining at the airport. The food was "meh" at best, but the company made up for it. Saying our goodbyes was bittersweet, especially when Grace insisted on being held by everyone at once. *Hold me everyone!* She has a way of making those moments feel extra special.

The flight back was a bit more... energetic, shall we say? Grace was having a hard time sitting still, so that first leg of the journey was a bit of a challenge. Fortunately, we had a layover where we didn't have to change planes, and by some miracle, she fell asleep sprawled across my lap and our row. I checked with the flight attendants, and they confirmed it wasn't a full flight. But then, a man came along and tried to claim one of our seats. I politely informed him that the plane wasn't full and suggested he find another spot (though I was really thinking, "If you wake her, I will lose my mind, Sir").

After landing we slowly got off the plane. Grace was half-asleep as we navigated through the airport on the way back, and by the time we reached the parking garage, she was done. We drove home, and she crashed right away, leaving me with a heart full of memories from our whirlwind day.

Would I do this experience again? Absolutely! Time with family, surprising my dad—there's nothing better. Plus, now Grace has a better understanding of what happens on an airplane, and I've learned that she can handle the travel … with a little help from snacks and naps.

Tips if you want to travel with a grandchild:

- If you're taking a young child on a day trip, pack plenty of snacks and activities—just know that you'll probably end up carrying most of it. If you're a parent, this is just standard operating procedure.
- Bring an empty water bottle to fill after security.
- Don't forget emergency medications, just in case.
- Tissues and wipes are lifesavers—pack them!
- If you're traveling with kids of different ages, bring activities they can do together to keep everyone entertained.
- Remember that no matter what happens, it's all part of the experience—laugh at the hiccups, and enjoy the ride.
- For the Phoenix Children's Museum, check online for discounts, and if you're local, consider a family membership. Also, bring wipes. Trust me on this one—you'll thank me later.

EXPERIENCE #2: LAUGHED MY WAY THROUGH IMPROV CLASSES

Experience #2: Sign-up for Improv Classes

I grew up doing drama and acting—oh, about 357 years ago. OK, maybe not that long, but it sure feels like a lifetime since I've been involved in anything theater-related. For the past couple of years, I've had this itch to dive back into that world, but I wanted to try something a little different this time around: improv. The idea of improv has always intrigued me—there's something a little daring about stepping into the unknown with no script, no plan, and just having to go with whatever comes your way. So, I decided to take the plunge and signed up for the January Level 1 Session at the Comedy Arena in McKinney, Texas. The class was six weeks long, and in the seventh week, we were going to perform on stage in front of a live audience. Gulp.

Our teacher, Ali, was a seasoned improv performer and a former schoolteacher, so she was brilliant at creating an environment where we could have fun and

"fail" (except in improv, there is no such thing as failure—
see, it's already a happy place). There were seven of us in
the class, all different ages and backgrounds. Two were
repeaters—not because they flunked, but because there
weren't enough people for a Level 2 class, so they came
back for more. There was a woman who owned a CPR
business and had survived a heart attack; she was all
about living life to the fullest, and improv was on her list.
Another classmate was a new mom, there was a young
guy with a ponytail, and one woman was a mom of not
one, but two sets of twins! Everyone had signed up for
different reasons—some to overcome anxiety, some for
fun, some to escape their children, and some just to meet
new people.

Each week, we learned a variety of improv games and
gradually worked our way up to short and long-form
improv. Let me tell you, it's not as easy as the pros make
it look, and it's definitely not the same as acting. In acting,
you have a script; you know what's coming next. In
improv, you have no idea what's coming. It's like opening
one door after another, not knowing what's on the other
side, but having to respond in some clever and funny way
while a room full of people watches. Yes, it can be a bit
nerve-wracking, but that's where the growth happens,
right?

The Comedy Arena also offers free tickets to their
shows while you're a student, as well as a weekly jam
session where all levels come together to play improv
games and practice short/long-form improv. I went to
one of these jam sessions with a good friend of mine who

had zero improv experience, and wouldn't you know it—he pretty much ruled. Some people are just naturals. Me? Not so much. But even though I "failed" spectacularly, I had an absolute blast, and that's what counts.

The night of our showcase arrived, and we all dressed in white shirts and jeans—a uniform of sorts, like the white belts in karate. I was nervous, especially since I had invited my daughter, granddaughter and a couple of friends to the show. I now had witnesses to my potential failure—no pressure, right? But here's the thing about improv: there's no such thing as messing up. It's all about those "yes, and" moments where you roll with whatever happens. We combined with a smaller class for our showcase, which added some extra energy to the room. We played different games, took suggestions from the audience, and just went for it.

I'm proud to report that I didn't make a total fool of myself, and most importantly, I had an absolute blast. Improv is basically playtime for adults, and we played our hearts out! I enjoyed it so much that I went on to take the Level 2 class, which was also a lot of fun. Although I'm not continuing for now (too many scheduling conflicts), it's definitely something I'd consider doing again in the future.

Would I do this experience again? Yes, and I did! I enrolled in Level Two the very next month.

Tips if you want to give improv a try:

- A lot of people think improv is just like acting, but it's actually all about play. It's so good for your brain to engage in creative play, and it keeps you sharp.

- People sign up for all kinds of reasons— whether it's to overcome anxiety, try something new, or just get out of the house. I highly recommend it to anyone considering it.

EXPERIENCE #3: DINED WITH YOUNG JEWISH PROFESSIONALS

I am Jewish. I am professional. I am, however, not young. But when I chose this activity, I selectively ignored that last part.

The program I joined is called Olami Dallas, which I found through a Facebook event. Only afterwards did I visit their website, which describes them as follows: "We are passionate about all things Judaism. Formerly YJP, and a branch of DATA, we are a community for 20-somethings (give or take a few years) Jewish young professionals in the Dallas greater area. Through learning, trips, and Jewish and social events we hope to help you share our passion. You only live once. Don't settle!"

Did you catch the "20-somethings" part? Yeah, I didn't either—until I showed up. Imagine a non-religious 49-year-old walking into a room filled with not only young people but also some dressed in traditional religious attire. To say I felt out of place would be an understatement. My Jewish involvement has been pretty minimal since my bat mitzvah. We observed the holidays growing up, but that was about it.

The theme of the night was the history of Jews in Persia (now known as Iran). Before the lecture began, we gathered in the kitchen to cook. And by "we," I mean mostly the women. The men were scattered about, chatting. As we cooked, I struck up a conversation with two really kind women who happened to be teachers. They were sharing their favorite TV shows, and I so badly wanted to jump in and talk about how much I loved *The Golden Bachelor* (a show about senior citizens dating), but I felt like that would've given away my age.

One of the women reminisced about the early 2000-2010 era, saying it was her favorite time. She then looked at me and asked, "That's when you were in high school, too, right?" Look, before I tell you how I answered, let me explain. I hadn't yet heard the lecture or eaten the food, so if I declared my age right then, I might've been booted out before the night even got started. So, and may my Jewish ancestors forgive me, I said, "Yes!" In theory, I was now playing the part of a young Jewish professional (improv came in handy).

Once the food was ready, we moved into the room for the lecture. The young rabbi gave an interesting talk about the history of Jews in Persia. Meanwhile, the nice guy sitting next to me asked if we could connect on social media. Oh boy. If I told him the truth, he'd find out I was a grandma among youth, an aged crasher at the party. So, I gave him my LinkedIn and hoped for the best.

After the lecture, we dined on the Persian food we had

prepared. One dish was an egg and herb concoction (someone got a bit heavy-handed with the salt), and the other was a meat stew. I've had good Persian food before —cooked by Persian people—and it was delicious. This, however, was made by a group of young professionals, and, well, let's just say it wasn't quite on the same level.

Would I do this experience again? No. Not because it wasn't great, but because it wasn't great when you're constantly self-conscious about being the oldest person in the room. I would, however, attend a similar event if it were for my age range or all age ranges – and if the food contained a little less salt.

Tips if you want to attend a religious-based event:

- First, check ahead of time what the topic is and whether it's age-appropriate for you.
- If you're not that religion, just let them know upfront.
- And if you're older, attend at your own risk!

EXPERIENCE #4: CACKLED AT A MASTER PANCAKE THEATER COMEDY SHOW

If you're fortunate enough to live near an Alamo Drafthouse theater, then you're in for a treat with this unique and entertaining experience. For over two decades, a comedy troupe out of Austin, known as Master Pancake Theater, has been hosting special events in movie theaters that offer a hilarious twist on film screenings. The concept is simple yet brilliant: they take a movie—anything from cult classics like *The Goonies* to obscure, low-budget flicks—and provide live, side-splitting commentary throughout the screening. I first experienced a similar Master Pancake Theater experience 10 years ago where the comedians brought in a movie they selected ahead of time (Goonies). So when I recently found out they were doing a twist to the event, I jumped at the chance to attend and dragged my good friend Liza with me.

So, what exactly is Master Pancake? The event is structured in a way that encourages audience participation and interaction, which adds to the fun. It starts with people from the audience bringing in DVDs of movies that they believe have the potential for some serious comedic roasting. These aren't your typical blockbuster hits but rather those "B" movies that never quite made it to mainstream success—often for good reason. The twist, however, is what makes this event so much fun.

Each person who brings a DVD gets 45 seconds on stage to pitch why their movie should be chosen for the evening's comedy spectacle. There's a lot of energy in the room as people cheer on their favorites, and through a process of elimination by audience applause, the selections are narrowed down to the top three. On the night I attended, the final decision came down to a dance-off, which only added to the chaotic and hilarious atmosphere. Ultimately, a movie called *Arcade* won the top spot. It was terribly horrible, which made it perfect.

With the winning DVD selected, the real magic of Master Pancake Theater kicked in. Three talented comedians took to the stage and began to riff on the movie, offering sharp-witted, off-the-cuff jokes and commentary that had everyone in the theater rolling with laughter. It was like a live improv show, but with the added twist of having a movie play out in the background—only to be mercilessly mocked. The humor was fast-paced and unpredictable, making it one of those experiences where you're constantly laughing and never quite sure what's going to happen next.

Would I do this experience again? Without a doubt!

Master Pancake Theater is based in Austin, so they don't often come up to Dallas, but now that I'm aware of their shows, I'm definitely planning to catch them whenever I can. The mix of live comedy and audience involvement creates a one-of-a-kind atmosphere that's hard to beat.

Tips if you want to go:

- If you can't make it to one of their live shows, you're in luck—some of their performances are streamed on Twitch, so you can enjoy the comedy from the comfort of your own home.
- Be ready to laugh! This isn't a typical movie-watching experience; it's a comedy show where the movie serves as the comedians' playground.
- If you're planning to bring a movie for the event, make sure to come prepared with a 45-second pitch to convince the audience why your selection should be the star of the night. However, if you just want to sit back and enjoy, that's perfectly fine, too—there's plenty of fun to be had as an audience member.

EXPERIENCE #5: FROZE MY BUNS OFF IN CRYOTHERAPY

If cryotherapy sounds like a cold and frosty adventure, you're right! This treatment involves immersing your body in extreme cold—around 10 degrees Fahrenheit, to be precise. The idea is that by exposing your body to such low temperatures, you can enjoy benefits like pain relief, reduced inflammation and even some potential weight loss. Although research is still catching up on these claims, it's an intriguing concept.

I was recovering from a recent back injury, so this seemed like the perfect time to give it a whirl. I managed to rope in my friend Andy, who was less than thrilled about the whole idea. Andy, being a doctor, had a particular aversion to the cold, and the biohazard sticker on the door didn't help ease his nerves.

Upon arrival, we were greeted by a room filled with recliners. Apparently, these are for targeted cryotherapy treatments. But we were gearing up for the full-body experience, which meant heading to a separate room.

In the cryotherapy chamber, everyone is required to wear gloves, socks and slippers, which the facility provided. I particularly enjoyed the dinosaur slippers—definitely a whimsical touch. Women are allowed to go all out (or rather, all in) with minimal clothing, while men have to keep on cotton underwear. Given that I was there with a friend, I opted to keep my short tank top and underwear on for modesty's sake.

Andy was the brave soul who went in first. He managed the full three minutes of the treatment, even though the technician suggested starting with 90 seconds for beginners. When my turn came, I had convinced myself that three minutes would fly by. Spoiler alert: it didn't. I barely made it to 90 seconds before tapping out. While my lower legs felt like they were in a freezer, the cold didn't quite reach my ailing back.

As part of the experience, we were also given algae tablets. I'm still not entirely sure how these supplements fit into the cryotherapy regimen, but they seemed like a good way to push some additional products.

Would I do this experience again? Maybe. I'm curious enough to try it for the full three minutes next time, provided my back and I are up for the challenge.

Tips if you want to try cryotherapy:

- **Dress appropriately:** Wear the provided gloves, socks and slippers. Enjoy the novelty of the dinosaur slippers!

- **Manage expectations:** Start with a shorter session (around 90 seconds) to gauge how you handle the cold.
- **Prepare for the cold:** Be ready for a chilling experience. It's cold, but that's the point!
- **Consider the supplements:** While not the main event, the algae tablets might be worth a try— just don't expect them to be the star of the show.

EXPERIENCE #6: JOINED A BAHAI FAITH MEANINGFUL CONVERSATIONS SESSION

I once had a college professor who belonged to the Bahá'í faith. She was incredibly kind, the type of person who made you feel regretful for even considering skipping class. Her warmth and compassion were infectious, and she had this uncanny ability to draw out the best in her students. I remember her sharing stories about her faith, emphasizing principles like unity and the importance of service to humanity. That was my introduction to Bahá'í: an ethos of kindness that stuck with me long after my college days ended. Fast forward a few years—OK, a few decades—and the only other thing I knew about it was what I'd read on the internet. So, when I stumbled upon an event on Facebook called "Meaningful Conversations," hosted by the Bahá'í community, I thought, "Why not?" At that time, only four people had RSVP'd, so I figured it would be an intimate little gathering. Spoiler alert: I was wrong.

Meaningful Conversations are held in various cities

across the country, providing a platform for open dialogue and connection. The session I attended was in a cozy coffee shop in Dallas, Texas. Picture it: a charming coffee house, dimly lit with twinkling fairy lights, the smell of freshly brewed coffee lingering in the air, and 25 people squeezed into a space meant for, well, maybe 15. It felt like a scene from a feel-good indie film—everyone buzzing with excitement and curiosity, eager to connect. But hey, we're all about togetherness, right?

The Facebook event description was delightfully vague, simply stating: "Spiritual conversations welcoming all perspectives in a search for the deeper truths that unite us." The theme of the evening was "Is Tolerance Enough?" Intriguing, right? So, naturally, I dragged a friend along—misery, or in this case, curiosity, loves company.

Upon arrival, we found the coffee shop closed to the public for the event. We grabbed a couple of chairs and joined the ever-expanding circle of participants. It started with about 15 people, but as the night went on, the circle grew to around 25. It was like the magic trick where clowns keep coming out of a tiny car, only less circus-y.

The rules were clear: no politics (thank goodness), and we were encouraged to embrace a loving posture of learning. Now, I wasn't entirely sure what a "loving posture" looked like, but I figured sitting up straight and smiling like I'd just won the lottery might be a good start. Maybe I'd even throw in a gentle nod, just to keep things lively.

We kicked off the evening with an icebreaker that felt like the perfect way to dive into the deep end. Going around the room, we shared our names and tackled the question, "In your view, what does it mean to not just tolerate someone, but to see them as yourself?" Talk about jumping into the ocean when you were expecting a leisurely dip in the kiddie pool! It was a bit daunting, but as the first person spoke, I could feel the tension lift. The answers that followed were thoughtful and varied, each one revealing a unique perspective on empathy and connection.

One person spoke of the importance of understanding another's story, while another emphasized the value of kindness in our interactions. You could see people really engaging, leaning forward in their chairs as if the very act of listening could somehow deepen their understanding. And of course, there were those who opted to pass—no shame in that! Sometimes, it's better to let your thoughts simmer before serving them up for everyone to digest.

As the conversation flowed, we transitioned to discussing nine principles from Bahá'í teachings, elegantly outlined in a pamphlet passed around like a prized party favor. Each principle aimed at uplifting humanity felt like a tiny spark of hope in a world that often seems overshadowed by division.

One principle that struck me deeply was the idea of regarding everyone as family. It was a comforting thought, like wrapping yourself in a cozy blanket on a chilly evening. But then my mind took a little detour— thank you, imagination! I envisioned Thanksgiving dinners with 7 billion relatives, each one vying for a seat at the table. Let's be real: that might be less of a feast and more of a chaotic food fight! I could almost hear the shouts of "pass the gravy!" echoing from the table.

Would I do this experience again? Absolutely! It's a great way to restore your faith in humanity (and maybe even snag a few new "family" members).

Tips if you want to go:

- Look up these groups on Facebook or Meetup —they're all over the country.
- Bring an open mind, a spirit of humility, and a willingness to scoot your chair over repeatedly to make room for new friends.

EXPERIENCE #7: SHOPPED SMART ON A GROCERY STORE TOUR WITH A DIETICIAN

Some people love using the grocery delivery service that became very popular during COVID. I, on the other hand, enjoy going to the grocery store. I like picking the avocados that don't look like dark green sagging breasts or exploring the sale items. However, it is not as exciting to do it in an Aldi discount store as it is in, say, Whole Foods. There is a grocery store chain here in Texas called Market Street. It is that magical place that straddles the line between "Wait, how much is this truffle oil?" and "I'm just here for the buy-one-get-one cucumbers." So, when I stumbled upon a dietitian-led food tour on Eventbrite, hosted by none other than Market Street, I knew it was time to elevate my grocery game. After all, who wouldn't want a free ticket to healthier living, one aisle at a time?

The tour promised 90 minutes of expert guidance on navigating the store's treasure trove of healthy options, with a little side dish of what-not-to-buy. It was like having a personal nutritionist in your shopping cart, minus the judgmental side-eye when you reach for that third box of cookies.

Leading our expedition was a registered dietician named Taylor, who had a unique talent for making nutrition sound less like a lecture and more like a cozy chat over a cup of (unsweetened, organic, and fair-trade) tea. Our merry band of seven (a mix of solos and couples) armed with reusable bags and a thousand questions, set off on this grocery journey like a pack of eager food adventurers. I was hoping for Costco sized samples on the way.

Our first stop? The bakery section, aka the land of temptation. Taylor didn't just walk us past the pastries; she practically performed a Jedi Mind Trick, suggesting that indulging doesn't have to turn into overindulging. She shared a brilliant tip: when the pastry cravings hit, opt for the bite-sized versions. That way, you can savor the sweetness without needing to unbutton your jeans afterward. Genius, right? It was like getting permission to have your cake and eat it too—just in smaller, waistline-friendly portions.

Next, we ventured into the ready-made meals area. Now, I know what you're thinking—pre-made meals? Aren't those just fast food in disguise? But hold your judgment! Taylor explained that these meals at Market Street are crafted with the input of dietitians. It's like having your personal chef, only without the messy kitchen and the awkward small talk. Knowing that your quick dinner has been given the nutritional thumbs-up? That's a win in my book.

Then came the cheese section—a place where dreams (and possibly cholesterol levels) are made. My personal heaven. Taylor gave us the inside scoop: when it comes to cheese, block is better. Why? Because shredded cheese often comes with a side of cellulose powder, which is basically sawdust in disguise. Yikes! So, for all the cheese lovers out there, grab a block and shred your way to a cleaner, less fibrous experience.

In the produce section, Taylor dropped a knowledge bomb that was equal parts enlightening and a little worrisome. Apparently, fresh produce can be a bit of a gamble for those undergoing chemotherapy due to the potential for germs. For these folks, canned or frozen veggies are a safer bet. Who knew that a can of green beans could be a lifesaver? She also preached the gospel of in-season produce and gave a shoutout to the locally-grown fruits and veggies from the great state of Texas. Support local farmers and eat fresher? Count me in!

Our journey continued to the seafood and meat section, where we waded into the farm-raised versus wild-caught debate. Taylor assured us that the nutritional differences are minimal, though the taste might swing one way or the other depending on your palate. And for all the protein buffs out there, here's a nugget of wisdom: chicken packs a bit more protein punch than beef. Plus, cooking in cast iron not only makes you feel like a gourmet chef but also ups the iron content in your meal. And if you want to be a real overachiever, pair your meat with citrus to enhance protein absorption. Talk about a dynamic duo!

Over in the milk section, including its dairy-free cousins, Taylor had some advice for postmenopausal women: steer clear of non-dairy milks with sunflower oils. As for regular milk, she sang the praises of Fairlife milk, with its high protein and low sugar content. She also emphasized the magic number for protein per meal: 20-30 grams. Suddenly, milk isn't just something you pour over cereal—it's a nutritional powerhouse.

Finally, we arrived at the bread aisle, where Taylor schooled us on the importance of fiber. She also shared the fascinating backstory of Dave's Killer Bread, which is not just delicious but also comes with a hefty dose of redemption. Founded by a former ex-con who now employs others with similar pasts, this bread is as good for the soul as it is for the body. Who knew bread could be so inspiring?

So, would I do this tour again? You bet your last organic banana I would. It wasn't just a grocery tour; it was a deep dive into the world of mindful shopping, and I walked away with a cartload of wisdom that's already changing the way I shop.

Tips if you want to go:

- Bring a notebook and pen because you're going to want to jot down all the golden nuggets of info Taylor drops. And if you've got specific questions, write them down ahead of time. This way, you'll be sure to squeeze every last drop of knowledge from the experience, just like that fresh-squeezed juice in aisle 7.

- If you don't have a Market Street in your area, contact your local grocery store and ask if they do tours.

EXPERIENCE #8: COOKED UP A COMPLETE MOROCCAN MEAL

Back in 2020, I had my heart set on a sun-soaked Greek adventure—imagine wandering ancient ruins, indulging in baklava, savoring blocks of feta cheese, and pretending I was in a scene from *Mamma Mia!* But, as with many grand plans that year, the pandemic decided to throw a wrench in the works. Greece would have to wait. Enter my friend Craig, who, sensing my travel blues, proposed an alternative: "Why don't you come over for Greek food?" Now, naturally, I assumed he meant *he* would cook for me while I lounged around awaiting the feast. But, oh no, Craig had a different idea—he meant we'd be cooking together. I was already halfway to hangry, and now this? Reluctantly, I agreed, unaware that this seemingly ordinary evening would kick off a tradition that would rival even the best of *My Big Fat Greek Wedding*.

That night, what started as a begrudging compromise

turned into the beginning of an epic culinary world tour. Craig and I, along with whoever else we could coax into joining our foodie escapades (rotating romantic interests included, of course), began our journey through the world's kitchens, one cuisine at a time. Our good friend Andy became a natural permanent sous chef. I was demoted to line cook (and rightfully so). We cooked our way through Jordanian, Senegalese, Spanish, Italian, French, German, Vietnamese, Thai, Eastern European, Irish, and Jewish dishes. We begin wearing costumes to celebrate the cuisine of the night. Each meal was a delicious excuse to bond, laugh and occasionally set off a smoke alarm. It was our cherished ritual until Craig's job took him across the pond to Ireland, leaving our culinary nights on a temporary hiatus.

Fast forward to the present—Craig's back in Texas, and so is our beloved tradition. Our trusty cooking partner Andy was ready to jump back into the fray, so we decided it was time to fire up the stove and rekindle the magic. This time, Andy suggested we take on Moroccan cuisine. He came armed with a menu from his favorite Moroccan restaurant, and Craig, who had a Moroccan friend, promised to bring the insider knowledge. The culinary challenge was set: pepper salad, tomato salad, meatball tagine, lentil soup (which, surprise, ended up with meat), and chicken Rfissa. It was the kind of menu that makes you want to loosen your belt before you've even started cooking.

As we began to cook, we quickly learned that

Moroccan cuisine is not for the faint of heart—or the light of spice rack. The real magic of Moroccan food lies in its complex spice blends, and let's just say our meatballs ended up tasting more like Nonna's Sunday special than anything you'd find in Marrakech. Clearly, our spice mix needed a little more Moroccan flair and a little less Italian grandma. The moral of the story? Spices are the secret to transporting your taste buds to far-off lands, and in this case, we might have missed the flight.

Would I do this experience again? Cooking nights with friends? You bet your tagine I would. It's the perfect way to bond, laugh and explore new cuisines without needing a passport. As for Moroccan food? Well, let's just say it's a bit like running a marathon—you're thrilled when it's over, proud of what you accomplished, but you might not be in a hurry to do it again. The prep was intense, but the experience was rewarding, even if I might opt for a slightly less demanding cuisine next time. Maybe next time we will focus on something that doesn't involve a spice cabinet explosion.

Tips if you're thinking of trying this:

- Invest in quality spices. Seriously, the right blend can make or break your dish and transport you straight to the bustling markets of Marrakech—or in our case, the trattorias of Italy.
- And if you can, rope in someone who knows their way around Moroccan cuisine. Having

Craig's insights saved us from a few rookie mistakes, and let's be honest, a little expertise goes a long way when you're dealing with dishes that have been perfected over centuries.

EXPERIENCE #9 WALKED THE CAMINO DE SANTIAGO PILGRIMAGE AND FOUND MYSELF

They say the Camino will give you what you need, and for me, this couldn't have been truer—or more profound. This. Was. So. Meaningful. The Camino de Santiago is a pilgrimage walk, but that doesn't quite capture the magic of it. According to the website Santiago Ways, it's a "collection of routes that lead to the Cathedral of Santiago de Compostela, traveled as a pilgrimage, usually on foot, as a way of paying homage to Saint James, whose remains rest in that temple." Back in the day, this journey was a deeply religious experience. These days, people walk the Camino for all sorts of reasons—adventure, life changes, grief, fun, exploration, hope and probably just a touch of insanity. But one thing is certain: the Camino is pure magic.

I first stumbled upon the idea of doing the Camino the year before COVID hit. I read somewhere that it took 40 days to complete, which is true if you start from France.

That little detail almost scared me off—who has 40 days? Not me. But after joining a few Facebook groups, I learned that you could do just a section of it, and as long as you walk 100km, you'll still get the certificate of completion. Suddenly, it felt doable, even for someone that didn't have a Moses amount of time to spare, like me.

I was interviewing for a job at that time. I knew I wanted to get in one more trip before the job started (spoiler alert: I didn't get the job). On my third interview, the hiring manager didn't show up. There was some type of miscommunication with the recruiter. So, this bought some time before the interview was scheduled. I booked my trip. I was going on a Camino.

Since it was so last minute, I had no time to train. Each day on the Camino you walk several miles (usually 10-12, but sometimes 20-25). About half the people carry their own backpack with them and the other half have their carryon transported to the next location. I had thrown my back out the month before, so I knew carrying my own backpack was a no for me. I spent three days planning the route I chose—the Portuguese Spiritual Route—booking hotels, planes, etc. And then, since I couldn't find a company to carry my bags since the hotels were out of the way, I changed my route. This meant losing money, but it also meant I wouldn't have to worry about my back. I chose the lighthouse route-Santiago de Compostela to Ferrieria to Muxia. All the other routes on the Camino end in Santiago where the cathedral is located. This route started there and ended at a lighthouse.

To begin my journey, I flew from Dallas to Madrid, where I had a long layover (which I used an upgrade to hang out in the airport lounge) before flying to Vigo, Spain. I was so exhausted that I went to bed at 7 p.m. Of course, this meant I woke up at 3 a.m., completely jet-lagged and confused. Vigo was supposed to be my starting point for the original Portuguese route, but since I had changed my plans, I had to stick with it because I already had a plane ticket there.

I digress. Waking up at 3 a.m. with no chance of falling back asleep, I decided to spend some time thinking about my intention for the Camino. I dedicated it to anyone who needed prayers. I posted a little video on Facebook, inviting people to reach out if they wanted to be on my Camino prayer list. The names came flooding in. It was truly touching and ended up being a great source of strength throughout my journey.

Since I was already awake, I waited for breakfast to open. This hotel did breakfast right! So much food, and they even had my favorite, tortilla de patata (Spanish omelette). After thoroughly enjoying breakfast, I walked a couple of miles, luggage in tow, to the train station. Vigo has this futuristic, Jetsons-like train station that just opened a few months ago. It looks like Saturn's rings. It was built because Vigo is such a hilly city, making it difficult for some people to climb to catch the train. Now, with escalators galore, it's much easier to use the trains. Brilliant engineering.

I hopped on the train to Santiago and sat next to an older gentleman who told me about his lady friend he was going to visit. Now, when I'm severely tired, my Spanish comprehension flies right out the window. So, jet-lagged as I was, his words turned to gibberish, and I could only smile and nod.

Upon arriving in Santiago, I was greeted by the guy who was transporting my luggage. It was such a relief to hand it off. I then walked the 25 minutes to the Cathedral. It was stunning, and since it was Good Friday, the place was packed with tourists and pilgrims alike. I made my way to the tourist office, which was buzzing with excitement, and picked up my Camino passport. The Camino Passport is what you get stamped as you walk, and you turn it in at the end to receive your certificate.

My first day was from Santiago to Alta de Pena, the longest stretch of my journey. Within minutes of starting, it began to pour. Fortunately, I came equipped with a thick raincoat and umbrella. The rain lasted about two hours before the sun made a brief appearance. That first day's walk was a doozy—20 miles, plus all the walking I had already done to get to and from train stations. I was not prepared. By the four-hour mark, my body was letting me know.

Now, I pride myself on being in shape. Before I left, I was teaching two Zumba classes and two Tabata classes a week. Cardio wasn't the issue; it was the constant walking motion for hours that my body wasn't ready for. My knees started to really hurt. Bad. I thought it would pass—it did not.

I came across a French woman sitting down with blisters. I offered her some Vaseline (a great trick to prevent blisters) but didn't sit down with her, worried that if I did, I wouldn't be able to get up again. A little while later, I saw a man in a car off the Camino route. It looked a bit suspicious, so I quickly answered his questions and kept walking. Later, I learned that his girlfriend and her two friends were walking the Camino, and he was supposed to go with them but had hurt his back, so he was driving alongside instead.

About 15 miles in, I was in major pain and ran into them again at a café. Wounded and humbled, I asked the boyfriend for help. He kindly drove me three miles ahead so I could limp the last two on foot.

I barely made it. I was in extreme pain. Along the way, I met a group of men from Portugal taking a Camino smoke break. They asked if I was okay, and I told them I was in pain but determined to keep going. Fifteen minutes later, they caught up to me (not a difficult feat since I was walking like a 90-year-old) and offered more help. One gave me ibuprofen, and then, out of pure mercy, the man put me on his back and carried me to the steps of my hostel. It was the embodiment of grace. I ate a little at the hostel and did everything I could for my knees —used my 10s unit, rubbed my legs, stretched—and went to bed.

The next morning, I was hopeful I could walk again. I was wrong. The pain was back in full force, and so was the rain. Day two was from A Pena to Abeleiroas. I found a walking stick that seemed like it had been carved just for me—Camino magic.

Several walkers passed me (not hard to do at my

pace), but many stopped to check on me. One gave me more ibuprofen, and later, a kind man gave me pain cream for my knees. Two women from Spain gave me one of their walking poles. Oh, the kindness of strangers!

Six hours into the walk, I stopped for lunch at a café with a fire going to dry off. I hung my socks to dry and chatted with another pilgrim. I desperately needed something to wrap my knees, but the local town didn't have a pharmacy, and the next town's pharmacy was closing in 30 minutes. It was already 2:30 p.m., and there was no way I could walk there in time. I called a taxi, and though we were worried the pharmacy might be closed, they kindly opened just for us. Camino magic, again.

I stocked up on supplies, limped to my apartment for the night, washed my clothes, grabbed a bite to eat, and went to bed.

There's rain, and then there's *windy rain*. You know what I mean? All week, it had been raining, but on this day, it was so windy that it would blow your Aunt Gertie (or her umbrella) away. I started walking but realized that it was not going to be safe to continue with the gusts. So, I made a tactical decision to call a taxi to take me to Lires, my next destination.

When I arrived in Lires, I checked into my small, charming hostel. It was rustic and cozy, just what I needed after battling the elements all week. I hung up my wet clothes and shoes to dry and decided to spend the day resting and reflecting. The rain continued, but I was grateful to be indoors, warm and dry. I ordered a hearty meal and, for the first time in days, felt my body relax.

The next morning, I woke up feeling much stronger, and the skies had cleared up a bit. My legs were still sore, but the sharp pain in my knees had dulled to a manageable level. This was the final stretch of my Camino journey, walking from Lires to Muxía. It wasn't a long walk, only about 15 kilometers (about 9 miles), and after everything my body had endured, I felt confident I could make it.

As I started out, the path was lined with beautiful wildflowers, and the fresh smell of rain still lingered in the air. I could see the ocean in the distance and knew that I was nearing the end of this part of my adventure. Along the way, I passed other pilgrims, some familiar faces and some new, and we exchanged nods of acknowledgment, all understanding the shared experience we were part of.

The sun finally came out as I neared Muxía, shining down as if to say, "You made it!" I felt a surge of pride and accomplishment. Reaching the end of the Camino at Muxía's lighthouse, where the waves crashed dramatically against the rocks, felt like the perfect end to this chapter of my life. I sat on a rock, staring out at the sea, reflecting on everything I'd learned along the way—the kindness of strangers, the resilience of my body, and the power of prayer and intention.

The Camino had tested me in ways I hadn't anticipated, but it had also given me so much more than I could've imagined. And in that moment, sitting by the ocean, I knew that every ache, every blister, every rainy mile had been worth it.

I stayed in Muxía that night, resting and enjoying the

little coastal town. The next morning, I took one last walk by the water, soaking in the tranquility before catching my bus back to Santiago. My Camino journey was over, but the memories, lessons and sense of peace I gained would stay with me forever.

Grateful. Tired. Reflective. Fulfilled. Changed.

Would I do this experience again? Yes! I would pick a new route to try and of course, I would train this time! It was such an impactful and beautiful experience.

Tips if you want to want to do it: So many tips, and I hope these will prove helpful for you if you decide to do a Camino. Here are my top 16 practical tips:

1. Wear the right shoes. Walk in them at least 20 miles before deciding if you will bring them or not. Also, pack a pair of waterproof sandals. They are helpful for showers and to air out your feet.

2. Train. Walk the amount of miles you are going to walk (build up to it) and wear your backpack with the exact weight you will be carrying. Look at the daily walk stretches for the Camino you will be walking.

3. Use a luggage transfer service if you don't want to carry a huge backpack. Keep in mind, for most of the carrier services, you have to know where you will end that day. So if you want to stop sooner, your luggage will be at the place you originally picked.

4. Buy and wear seamless socks. Godsend! Practice in socks, too, so you can get a feel for how they do long-term. I bought Blister Resist socks and Dang Tough Socks (both on Amazon).

5. Vaseline and trimmed toenails for your feet. Put on Vaseline every morning at any potential hot spots for blisters. It will save you!

6. Look up the weather before you go and pack accordingly. Think layers. I went in April. I was really glad to have an umbrella and a multi-layered jacked that was a rain jacket. I also packed a poncho for the really rainy day. I also packed sunscreen and a wooly hat.

7. Self-care for the end of the day: sports tape, ibuprofen, massage cream.

8. Walking poles. You can buy these when you get there and lots of Pilgrims give them away after their walk since you can't take them on the plane.

9. Know your sleep ability and if needed, book a private room. If you sleep in a community room, someone will snore. I booked private rooms throughout my whole Camino.

10. Consider using apps to help Camino Ninja and Buen Camino to help you on your trails.

11. Join a Camino Facebook group to help get tips for your specific Camino.

12. Bring a journal to write your journey and to take notes.

13. Bring a charger—one for the room and one for your walk.

14. Use a company like Wise to have Euros pre-loaded on a card (this is for anyone not living in a country with Euros).

15. Use stretch videos before and after each walk DAILY. YouTube is helpful for this.

16. Take some snacks with you and bring a fillable water bottle that you can take with you each day.

EXPERIENCE #10: INDULGED IN A MEAL AT A MICHELIN STAR RESTAURANT

Calling all foodies—this one's for you! For years, visiting a Michelin Star restaurant has been on my bucket list. If you're not familiar with Michelin Stars, here's a tasty tidbit from USA Today: A Michelin Star restaurant is a dining spot that's been awarded one or more stars by the Michelin Guide, a prestigious and globally recognized rating system. The guide evaluates restaurants based on several criteria, including ingredient quality, cooking mastery, flavor, value for money and consistency.

Here's what those stars actually mean:

- **One Star:** A very good restaurant in its category, offering cuisine prepared to a consistently high standard.
- **Two Stars:** Excellent cooking that's worth a detour. The restaurant serves skillfully crafted dishes of outstanding quality.

- **Three Stars:** Exceptional cuisine that's worth a special journey. The restaurant offers remarkable dishes that are meticulously executed and deliver a unique dining experience.

Receiving a Michelin Star is a major culinary accolade, often leading to increased prestige and business for the restaurant.

Now, back to the experience. While I was in Spain for the Camino, I discovered that there are plenty of Michelin-starred restaurants there (though not all of them boast stars). Texas doesn't have any, as there's no Michelin chapter there yet, but you can find some in New York, California, Colorado and Illinois. To celebrate the end of my Camino, I decided to try one in Santiago de Compostela.

The place was called Casa de Marcelo. It was a charming little restaurant decked out in red and white— kind of an Italian vibe, though the cuisine was distinctly Spanish. When I walked in, they seated me at the bar (food counter), took my jacket and backpack, and I suddenly had three servers at my disposal. There was only one other couple in the restaurant, and after my solo Camino, I was eager to chat about the food. Unfortunately, I soon discovered that the couple spoke no English. We ended up using sign language, which for me meant a lot of Spanish miming. They were incredibly sweet, and it was amusing to see us all making "thumbs-up" gestures and "mmm" sounds.

The meal began with a mocktail that was out of this world—cucumber with sweet syrup and some secret magic. Delicious! Next came a piece of wet bread with pesto sauce—interesting, but not the highlight. The in-house made bread was far better. Then came cold soup with Galician clams in corn and coconut, followed by oysters and mussels in lemon foam served on what I thought was rice but turned out to be coarse salt. My spoonful of salt was a surprise! And not the good kind!

Then, an avocado half was served, filled with fresh bull crab and sea urchin, topped with green sauce. It was face-down, so cutting into the avocado revealed the treasures inside. Delicious! Next up was shrimp mousse with finely chopped portobello mushrooms—pure drool-worthy goodness. Squid in corn cream with fish ink and croutons followed, and though squid isn't my favorite, it was surprisingly good. Fish in broth over potato came next—so fresh! Finally, dessert time! I chose green tea macarons stuffed with lemon sorbet. You had to smack it with your spoon to eat it. They topped it off with a layered filo dough dessert with cream between each layer and a candle for my birthday.

Each portion was small—maybe two to five bites worth—but just enough to savor every mouthful. It was fascinating to watch the kitchen team respectfully supporting each other. At the end, I asked to get a picture of the chef, and he called everyone in for the shot. It was a delightful experience with incredible service. I spent $147 on the meal, and every bite was worth it.

Would I do this again? Yes! A thousand times yes! Foodgasm for the win!

Tips for your Michelin adventure: If you're heading to a city with Michelin restaurants, be sure to book a reservation ahead of time—they fill up fast, especially on weekends.

EXPERIENCE #11: EXPLORED THE CHARM OF SANTIAGO DE COMPOSTELA, SPAIN

Ah, Santiago de Compostela! The grand finale of the Camino de Santiago, and boy, does it live up to the hype. After walking my way through the Camino in reverse (yep, I like to do things a bit differently), I was ready to dive into this city and explore all it had to offer.

Santiago de Compostela isn't just famous for its religious significance—it's a tourist hotspot, and for good reason. Nestled in the heart of Galicia in Northern Spain, this city is like a treasure trove of history and culture, with the magnificent cathedral taking center stage.

So, here's a little history for you from Google: The legend of Santiago de Compostela is deeply tied to St. James the Greater, one of Jesus's apostles. After Christ's resurrection, St. James embarked on a mission to the Iberian Peninsula (now Spain and Portugal). He was martyred by beheading around 44 AD, and his remains were miraculously transported back to Spain by his followers. Fast forward to the ninth century, and a hermit named Pelayo rediscovered his tomb, marked by a starry field. Hence, "Compostela" (Campus Stellae or Field of Stars). Voilà, Santiago de Compostela became a pilgrimage hotspot, second only to Jerusalem and Rome.

The Cathedral of Santiago de Compostela, a masterpiece of Romanesque architecture with some Gothic and Baroque bling, is the city's crown jewel. It's not just a big church; it's the spiritual epicenter of the city and the end goal for many a weary pilgrim.

I had just one day to soak in the sights, so I kicked off my adventure at the local farmer's market. This wasn't your run-of-the-mill market with the occasional fruit stand and a bunch of Etsy crafts. No, this was a full-blown food extravaganza. There were tunnels of seafood, meat, bread, cheeses and, of course, a rainbow of fruits and veggies. I treated myself to avocado toast on the freshest bread I've ever tasted and scored some cheese at a stand that felt like it was plucked straight from a foodie's dream.

Next up was the main square in front of the cathedral. I hopped on a tram for a city tour, complete with headphones. The English translation? Let's just say it was a bit of a linguistic adventure. Despite that, the tour was a blast. Santiago is a sprawling city with parks, a large university campus, museums and bustling streets.

After the tram ride, I took a leisurely stroll through Alameda Park. It's a charming spot where you can enjoy views of the cathedral while people-watching—families strolling, runners jogging and teenagers sneaking in some smooches. Classic park vibes!

Would I do this experience again? Absolutely! I hope to lace up my walking shoes for another Camino someday and return to this vibrant city.

Tips if you want to do it:

- Spain's "Medio Día" means everything shuts down from 1:30 to 3 p.m. Only bars and restaurants keep their doors open. Plan accordingly!
- There are several Michelin Star restaurants in Santiago, so if you're a foodie, look them up.
- Museum buffs, you're in luck—there are plenty. For those like me who aren't as museum-inclined, Google will be your best friend.

EXPERIENCE #12: PEEKED INTO THE MAGIC OF PORTO, PORTUGAL

Have you seen those captivating photos of Porto? You know, the ones with the flat, colorful houses that seem to tumble down the hillside along the river? Porto had been on my travel wish list for as long as I can remember. So, when I found myself just a stone's throw away in Santiago de Compostela, I couldn't resist the temptation to visit. However, I had only one day—well, to be honest, about three hours. I highly recommend giving yourself a bit more time if you're planning to explore Porto.

My journey to Porto was a bit of an adventure. I walked 20 minutes from my hotel to the train station, took an hour-long train ride to Vigo, Spain, and then hopped on a 2-hour bus to Porto. Arriving at Porto's airport, I still needed to navigate the metro (subway) to get downtown. All in all, my travel time added up to eight hours. So, my advice? Don't try to squeeze all this into a single day if you can avoid it!

During my marathon journey, I did a little research

and stumbled upon a walking tour itinerary. Porto is famously hilly—picture steep inclines that make every day feel like a glute workout. The itinerary recommended starting at the top and working your way down. So, I took the metro to Jardem de Morros, a stunning park perched high above the city. By the time I arrived, my bladder was practically bursting. After hours of traveling, I found that the nearby bathroom was out of order. I tried hotels and other businesses, but no luck. Finally, I found a bakery, bought a Pastel de Nata (custard pastry) and a fried cod cake just to get the key to their restroom. Early tip: Keep a stash of Euro coins for bathrooms or small purchases.

With that challenge behind me, my tour officially began. Jardem de Morros offered panoramic views of Porto and the iconic De Louis Bridge. It was a breathtaking sight and a must-see. The park was alive with tourists and locals enjoying the day, making it a perfect starting point for exploring Porto.

From there, I started my descent down the incredibly steep hill, surrounded by vibrant street vendors and entertainers. Porto is bursting with energy! The buildings are adorned with colorful tiles, creating a dazzling visual feast. As I reached the riverfront, I was greeted by throngs of tourists, bustling restaurants and numerous boat tour vendors. Although I didn't have time for a riverboat tour, it's something I'd definitely consider on a return visit.

I was eager to try Porto's famous sandwich, the Francesinha. This hearty creation is essentially a meaty grilled cheese extravaganza layered with bread, cheese, ham, fresh sausage, pork sausage, veal steak and sometimes topped with a fried egg (mine didn't come with the egg). It's then smothered in a rich sauce that, to my taste, resembled Campbell's tomato soup mix. It wasn't exactly a culinary revelation, but I'm glad I gave it a shot—trying local specialties is part of the adventure!

With about an hour left before catching the metro back to the bus station, I wandered through Porto's old town. The architecture and ambiance reminded me of a blend of Paris, Barcelona and New York. I also explored the newer parts of the city, which, though modern, still retained a certain old-world charm. On the crowded metro ride back to the airport, I struck up a conversation with a friendly psychotherapist from Argentina. We chatted about mental health, pandemic life and everything in between.

After making a final restroom stop at the airport, I boarded my bus back to Vigo. But, surprise! Vigo has two train stations. I arrived at the wrong one, and after a frantic search with another traveler, we missed our train by just a minute. We had to buy new tickets and wait an additional hour. We made the best of it by grabbing a drink (water for me, beer for her) at a nearby bar.

By the time I returned to Santiago, I was exhausted but satisfied. Porto was every bit as beautiful as the postcards had promised.

Would I do this experience again? Absolutely! I'd love to return and spend a couple of days there, and explore the Douro Valley as well.

Tips if you want to do it: Don't try to see Porto in just four hours. Take your time, go on a tour and spend a few days there if possible.

- Indulge in all the local food you can handle, make time for the street performers and definitely consider a river cruise.
- Use the metro to navigate the city efficiently. Porto's old town is spectacular, but the rest of the city is sprawling, so plan accordingly.

EXPERIENCE #13: TRAVELED TO A CORUNA, SPAIN FOR A TASTE OF THE COAST

We've all heard about Barcelona and Madrid—Spain's flashy, big-name cities—but there's something truly magical about its smaller towns and cities. A Coruña, for example, is a gem you might not have on your radar, but trust me, it's worth a visit. Located just a quick 30-minute train ride from Santiago de Compostela, A Coruña was my chosen spot for my last full day in Spain before jetting off to Madrid. And oh boy, was it the perfect choice!

Upon arrival, I was stunned by the city's sheer size. It's a bustling port town that seamlessly blends the old with the new. And get this: it boasts Europe's oldest running lighthouse! This iconic structure is surrounded by a field of yellow wildflowers, standing guard over both the town and the sea. The coastal walk offers stunning views, though be warned: the wind is relentless. It felt like nature's way of giving me a free facial exfoliation.

Desperate for shelter from the wind, I ducked into a

cozy bar/restaurant. Time for tapas! I indulged in some Russian salad with a side of bread, which was as delightful as it sounds. But why stop there? I decided to seek out more pinchos—essentially tapas' smaller, even more delightful cousins.

In the old city, I found a charming spot where I ordered croquettes (little fried morsels of happiness stuffed with anything from potatoes to seafood), a fresh green salad and flatbread topped with cheese and caramelized onions. Just as I was savoring my meal on the patio, the skies opened up and rain came pouring down. I moved my table so that the neighboring patrons could stay dry, while a street vendor selling an array of knick-knacks tried to shield himself from the deluge. I invited him to join me and share my food, but he politely declined, explaining that he was fasting for Ramadan.

The vendor, hailing from Africa, was in Spain to support his family back home. He had come to earn money to send to his wife and child, navigating a three-year wait to work legally. His knick-knacks were his lifeline. I packed up my leftovers and sent them with him —a small gesture that felt deeply rewarding.

With the rain easing, I continued my exploration. I visited the Mayor's Palace and indulged in some pastries —yes, it was one of those days where calories don't count. I wandered by the pier, hoping for a glimpse of the house owned by the Zara Founder Amancio Ortega Gaona (the clothing store mogul) but no luck. Still, the view was worth the stroll. I also discovered that Picasso's father hailed from A Coruña—small world!

The city was alive with families, friends and couples strolling the streets. Spain has this enchanting quality of making everyday scenes seem extraordinary.

My day wrapped up with a sprint to catch my train, followed by a quick dash to the bus stop. I opted for the euro bus instead of the 30-euro taxi, a choice I later regretted as the bus was late and I barely made it to the airport in time. But hey, I made it, and I'm grateful for the chance to explore this charming city.

Would I do this experience again? Absolutely! A Coruña deserves more than just a fleeting visit.

Tips if you want to do it: Take the train for a quick and scenic ride. Explore the old city and the pier, and don't miss the lighthouse. And remember to wear a windbreaker—unless you're aiming for that free exfoliation experience.

EXPERIENCE #14: EXPLORED JOHREI ENERGY HEALING AND DISCOVERED MY ZEN

Every few months, a Holistic Fair makes its way to my area, and it's like a mini-vacation for my soul. I dive headfirst into yoga classes, indulge in sound baths and explore various vendors hawking everything from crystals to handcrafted soap. This year, I roped in my friend Kristi for the journey. We meandered through booths, soaking up the peace and positive vibes, until we stumbled upon a curious setup in the middle of the room —Johrei Energy Healing.

Johrei, for those who aren't familiar, is a Japanese healing technique that piqued our interest. According to the practitioners, it involves channeling healing energy from one person to another, supposedly to restore balance and well-being. Intrigued, we decided to give it a whirl.

We were guided to a circle of chairs and instructed to sit comfortably, hands folded right over left, palms facing up. The leader explained that in Japan, Johrei practitioners stand before you, and their energy flows into your head to heal your energy. Kristi and I braced ourselves for some sort of mystical touch or head-honoring ritual. We followed directions dutifully, closing our eyes and preparing for what we imagined might be a deeply transformative experience.

Halfway through, we were told to lower our heads. Expecting a gentle touch or perhaps some kind of energy transfer, we kept our eyes shut, ready to feel the magic. Instead, the session wrapped up with the leader cheerfully announcing, "OK, we're finished!" and presenting us with bags of rice. Yes, rice. It wasn't exactly the crystal or talisman I'd envisioned, but it was a pleasantly surprising end to our session.

I cooked the rice a few days later, and I must say, it was excellent—fluffy, flavorful and perfect alongside chicken. So, while the spiritual benefits of Johrei were a bit elusive, the rice was a tangible and delicious takeaway.

Kristi, ever the inquisitive soul, struck up a conversation with the practitioner. She learned that Johrei is based on the idea that the healing light flows from the practitioner to the recipient. It's a poetic and serene concept, but despite the beautiful philosophy, neither Kristi nor I felt any noticeable shift in our energy. However, we did leave with a smile and a newfound appreciation for a good bowl of rice.

Would I do this experience again? Probably not. While it was a fascinating glimpse into a different healing practice, it didn't leave a lasting impact on me. However,

I'm grateful for the rice and the chance to explore something new.

Tips if you want to try it:

- Embrace the rice. Seriously, GET. THE. RICE. It's a surprising treat!
- For more information on Johrei and its practice, check out their website at https://www.johrei.org . If you're curious about energy healing or just looking for a unique experience, it's worth a look.

EXPERIENCE #15: ATTEND A SÉANCE AND DIDN'T GET HAUNTED

Did you ever use a Ouija board at a slumber party as a kid? You know, the one that supposedly summoned spirits to answer your burning questions, like "Does Brian like me?" (Spoiler: Brian did not, despite the board's enthusiastic "yes.") The thrill of the unknown was always tantalizing. So, naturally, I wanted to explore a séance and see if I could finally get some cosmic clarity about Brian's feelings—or perhaps just indulge in a bit of spooky fun.

I found a séance happening at Entelechea in Richardson, Texas, just a 20-minute drive from my place. Entelechea offers quite the metaphysical buffet: community space, free Wi-Fi, a reading nook, a meditation room and various practitioners offering services like sound healing and reiki. The séance was held in a cozy backroom and set me back $20—a small price for a slice of the supernatural.

Arriving at the venue, I discovered that I was one of the early birds. The room had a circle of chairs, and I settled in while scrolling through my phone. Soon enough, the room filled up to about 15 participants. The psychic, our guide to the great beyond, made her entrance and threw a few electric cat toy balls onto the floor. These were the kind that light up and roll around, meant to captivate a feline's attention. Apparently, they also serve as spirit communication devices. Who knew?

The séance was designed to be a loving experience, aimed at connecting with deceased loved ones. If you weren't feeling the vibe, you could simply say "no thanks," and the spirits would gracefully exit stage left. The psychic began with a heartfelt message for two sisters in their 60s, whose deceased brother seemed to be making quite the impression, especially regarding guitars. The sisters were visibly moved and excited by the personal message.

Then, it was my turn. The psychic channeled my grandmother, who, according to the séance, was all about her independence and apparently had some strong opinions about my dad's behavior. I had to chuckle because this was so out of character for the sweet, loving grandma I knew. It was like the spirit world had mixed up their files. After that, I found myself eyeing the cat balls for a bit of entertainment (and not just because they were designed for our feline friends).

Many participants were there seeking closure from their departed relatives, and it was heartening to see a few people finding some peace. One young woman insisted that she was also receiving messages from the other side. The leader was kind and patient, doing her best to reassure everyone.

The whole experience lasted about two hours, and I have to admit, my bladder was starting to send distress signals. I bumped into a fellow participant afterward who was equally baffled by her reading. She'd had a few sessions with this psychic and mentioned that the last two readings left her "thinking." AKA—The reader was way off the mark.

Would I do this experience again? Sure, why not? It was an intriguing venture into the unknown, though it's not at the top of my list. I have a friend who's keen on going, so I might tag along for another round.

Tips if you want to try it:

- Go in with zero expectations and keep an open mind (not because you necessarily believe in it, but so you're not judgmental). It's helpful to know what type of séance you're attending— some can be more intense or serious, while others, like this one, are designed to be gentle and loving.
- Oh, and if they offer cat balls, don't forget to appreciate their dual purpose and offer a silent meow.

EXPERIENCE #16: REVAMPED MY WARDROBE WITH A CLOTHING STYLIST

Are you a shopper? Let me be honest—I'm not. Before the pandemic, my wardrobe was a hodgepodge of comfy pieces, and since then, I've practically lived in yoga pants and tank tops. But imagine my delight when I discovered you can meet with a professional stylist at Nordstrom for FREE. Yes, you read that right—no need to fork out a fortune for a fashion diva. Just hop online, schedule an appointment, and your very own style expert will be ready to revamp your look.

So, on a quest for a wardrobe refresh, I booked an hour-long session. The process was simple: you pick what you need—be it new work attire, exercise gear, a special occasion outfit or a complete wardrobe overhaul. You set a budget, share any style inspirations, and voilà, a stylist is assigned to you.

I was excited but also a tad apprehensive. My goal was to step out of my comfortable gym wear and into something a bit more polished. When I arrived at

Nordstrom, my stylist, Yvette, was already busy putting together workout clothes for me. I had to chuckle; I've amassed enough gym wear to open my own boutique, so I was ready for something a bit different. With that, we embarked on a mini fashion adventure through the store away from active gear.

Yvette, a 22-year-old art student with an impeccable eye for style, had some creative ideas. I'll admit, some of her selections made me think, "Are you sure about this?" But as we sifted through racks of clothes, her choices began to grow on me. We explored the shoe department, browsed the purse section, and even glanced at the jewelry, making the whole experience feel like a personal fashion tour.

Then came the fitting room drama. There were definite hits—outfits that made me feel like a million bucks—and a few misses. PSA: If you're accustomed to Walmart sizing, prepare for a reality check at Nordstrom. And those prices! For a gal used to the clearance racks at Ross, the price tags were a shocking revelation. It felt like I was shopping in a different currency. After some serious deliberation (and a bit of sticker shock-induced vertigo), I settled on a stunning dress and a pair of shoes that, while pricey, were absolutely fabulous.

To ease the post-shopping shock, I decided to swing by TJ Maxx on my way home. After Nordstrom, everything there felt like a steal! I ended up finding a whole array of new clothes—yes, for the price of that one dress from Nordstrom. Naturally, I had to return the dress (though I did adore it), but I felt like I'd made the right choice.

In the end, I walked away with a pair of $55 shoes from Nordstrom, which felt like a small victory. More importantly, I learned a lot about fashion trends and how to adapt them to a more budget-friendly shopping strategy.

Would I do this experience again? Absolutely! But next time, I'd make sure my budget could keep up with my shopping aspirations.

Tips if you want to give it a try:

- Know your budget and what you need for your wardrobe before setting foot in the store.
- Book your appointment on Nordstrom's website.
- Be prepared to splurge a little, but remember, you can use the stylist's suggestions as inspiration and find less expensive alternatives elsewhere.
- Have fun with the experience! Whether you end up buying a whole new wardrobe or just a couple of standout pieces, it's a great way to shake things up and get a fresh perspective on your style.

EXPERIENCE #17: FLOWED MY WAY THROUGH A TAI CHI LESSON

I grew up watching the Karate Kid. Remember Ralph Macchio? Oh, the teenage dreams of swooning over the Karate Kid! Maybe that's why Tai Chi popped into my head as a new experience to try. Or maybe it was just my curiosity about why people practice this slow-motion exercise and whether it could really be good for you.

I began my search to find a Tai Chi class near me. Despite being in a bustling Dallas metroplex, there weren't many options that fit my schedule. Eventually, I found Cheng Ming USA in Plano, Texas. The trial class was $30—outside my typical gym budget, but a good price for a one-time try. The reviews raved about Eric, the owner, so I decided to give it a shot.

On a Tuesday evening, I arrived a bit early to settle in and pay (yes, I brought a check because they didn't accept credit cards). Eric greeted me warmly, and I was met by two other women waiting for the class. We started chatting, and it turned out we were all in our 50s. They looked fantastic, which was a promising endorsement for Tai Chi.

Tai Chi is a unique blend of very slow self-defense movements designed to connect the Chi (energy) with the body's meridians for enhanced flow and health. It's part meditation, part movement (and did I mention very slow movement?). It helps with balance, organ health, and mental wellness. Honestly, when was the last time you saw an angry person practicing Tai Chi? Exactly.

The class started with stretching. There were about 15 of us, mostly in my age group or older. Eric took a seat at a desk to read a book, while one of the participants, a man in his 70s, led us through the stretches. He shouted "hi" each time we moved to a new stretch. He noticed I was new and made sure to guide me with his eyes, which was kind and helpful (and sometimes a little intimidating).

After stretching for about 15 minutes, we split into two groups. Eric asked if we wanted to practice 1 or 2 moves or join the group for a full Tai Chi practice. I opted for the full 30-minute session. There were no more "hi" shouts, but the group smoothly transitioned through the moves and sequences. It felt like being in a slow-motion karate video. With no prior experience, I just followed along, like a student who was accidentally placed in an advanced class (read: totally lost but pretending I was not). I struggled to keep up but felt a bit more in control of my body and calm by the end.

Eric came over to compliment my effort, and though I chuckled, I appreciated his encouragement. He's been practicing Tai Chi for forty years, so I'm sure I wasn't the first beginner to dive in headfirst. I also met his mother, who has been practicing Tai Chi since 1976. Seeing someone move so gracefully in their 80s was inspiring. Additionally, the older men in the class demonstrated remarkable flexibility, suggesting that Tai Chi truly benefits aging bodies.

I spoke with another woman who seemed like a Tai Chi pro. She had been practicing for a year and a half, attending classes three times a week. She loved how Tai Chi improved her balance, body awareness, and even provided an internal organ massage. She also mentioned that the type of Tai Chi we practiced was Cheng Ming, with other styles like Qi Chong being more meditative and slower. Tai Chi's benefits, especially for aging, are indeed impressive.

Would I do this experience again? Absolutely. Tai Chi has intrigued me, especially with its focus on balance as we age. Plus, the class following ours used wooden sticks, which seemed intriguing—though I'd need to be careful not to poke anyone by mistake.

Tips If You Want to Try It

- Research Different Styles: Look up various Tai Chi styles, like Cheng Ming or Qi Chong, to find one that resonates with you.
- Start with a Beginner's Class: Opt for a beginner-friendly class or private instruction to get personalized guidance and ask questions without interrupting the flow.

- Prepare for Quiet: Tai Chi is a calm and quiet practice, so be ready to absorb information visually and adjust to the slow pace. If you have questions, it's best to ask before or after the class to avoid disrupting the serene environment.

EXPERIENCE #18: ROAD TRIPPED TO FREDERICKSBURG, TX WITH FRIENDS

Ah, the magic of a Girls' Trip! There's nothing quite like the camaraderie, laughter and occasional misadventure that comes with traveling with the right friends. Fredericksburg, Texas, had been on my radar for years, so when it became the chosen destination for our latest girls' getaway, I was thrilled. And let me tell you, it did not disappoint!

Nestled in the heart of Texas, Fredericksburg is the state's very own wine country. It's relatively close to Austin and boasts over 60 wineries. The town has become a hotspot for bachelorette parties, anniversary celebrations and weekend escapes, so we decided to join the throngs and make it our destination.

So, who's in this "we" I keep mentioning? It's me, Priscilla, Gaby and Rachel—all of us bonded through our Zumba classes many moons ago. Priscilla, a busy mom and business owner, was especially ecstatic since this was her first getaway from her kids since, well, their birth (the oldest is now 13). Rachel had been dreaming of visiting Fredericksburg, and Gaby, who had been there before, was our resident expert.

After a five-hour drive from Dallas, we arrived at our Airbnb around 11:30 p.m. In our sleepy state, we managed to accidentally punch the code into the wrong house. Not exactly the welcome committee you want in Texas! Luckily, we avoided any unwanted confrontations.

Our actual Airbnb, a mere three houses down, was charming and perfect. Pri and I had our own rooms, while Gaby and Rachel, being self-proclaimed snorers, shared a room (we planned ahead on that one). Priscilla, ever the prepared one, was walking around the house with a strange red light. Turns out, she was checking for hidden cameras. And yes, she brought two guns along for added security, courtesy of her well-meaning husband. My only request was not to accidentally shoot me if I made a midnight dash for the kitchen.

The next morning, we kicked off our day with breakfast at Sunset Grill and then strolled through the downtown area. It was predictably hot (hello, Texas!), but the town was adorable, with plenty of quirky shops and eateries. A visit to the visitor center revealed not just a bounty of wineries but also peach farms. As the sole nondrinker in the group, I was all about the peaches! We had also pre-booked a hike at Enchanted Rock, so that adventure was on the horizon.

We visited several wineries—maybe 7 or 8?—including one with a rhino (yes, an actual rhino) and another with a massive wedding venue. One winery was super laid-back with cornhole games. Fredericksburg truly has something for everyone!

Post-winery, we ventured to the peach farm. Although they were out of peach ice cream (heartbreaking!), we scored some juicy peaches and fresh berries. We then decided to dress up for dinner, so off we went to Walmart. I ended up with two super cute dresses and, shockingly, more gym clothes. Because who doesn't need more workout gear?

Enchanted Rock was a highlight, though the weather was a challenge. It was incredibly windy and, did I mention? Hot. Like, really hot. If you're planning to hike there, make sure you're somewhat experienced and armed with plenty of water. We completed our trek, but then it was straight back to the AC for some much-needed relief.

For dinner, we hit Hill and Vine, where the food was good, but the service was even better. We capped off the day with a Netflix binge—because, why not?

Would I do this experience again? Absolutely! I'd love to visit Fredericksburg again, preferably in the spring or fall when the weather is a bit kinder.

Tips if you want to try it:

- **Book ahead for Enchanted Rock:** You'll need reservations, so plan ahead and go in the morning if it's hot.
- **Stay hydrated:** Bring plenty of water; it can get scorching!

- **Dress the part:** Many folks were decked out in cute outfits and dresses, while we stuck with gym clothes. Comfort is key!
- **Check out wine tastings in town:** If you prefer to stay local, many shops offer tastings.
- **Visit the Visitor Center:** They provide fantastic recommendations on which wineries to explore.

EXPERIENCE #19: FOWLED AROUND AT THE BOWLING LIKE GAME OF FOWLING

If you've ever wondered what happens when you mix bowling, football and cornhole, then you're about to meet your new favorite game: Fowling. Born in the tailgating paradise of Detroit, Mich., Fowling is as much about fun and creativity as it is about knocking down pins with a football. According to the lore, this brainchild of Chris Hutt and his friends started with a failed attempt to build a bowling alley at the Indianapolis 500. When that didn't quite pan out, they gave themselves an "F" for effort. But as fate would have it, during one of their tailgates, someone accidentally rolled a football over a set of bowling pins, sparking the idea that would become Fowling. And thus, the Fowling Warehouse was born. It has since spread to eight cities, mostly in the Midwest, proving that football and bowling make for a fantastic mix.

When a Fowling location opened near me, I was intrigued but never quite got around to visiting—until, of course, a date opportunity presented itself. My date asked what fun things there were to do in the area, and like a lightning bolt of inspiration, the Fowling Warehouse popped into my mind.

So what's the deal with Fowling? Imagine two sides, each with a set of 10 bowling pins. You stand on one side and hurl a football with the goal of knocking down the pins on the opposite side. We're not talking about plastic pins here—these are the real deal, so you've got to put some serious muscle behind those throws. Given that my throwing prowess is, well, nonexistent, I was prepared for a challenging game. My date, on the other hand, had an arm like a cannon. Unfortunately, even his impressive throws didn't guarantee success. Turns out, there's a mysterious element to Fowling that neither of us could quite crack.

Realizing that neither of us were going to be the next Fowling champions anytime soon, we decided to make our own rules (since we weren't entirely sure of the original ones anyway). We moved to one side and took turns throwing the football, with the winner being whoever knocked down the last pin. I managed to win once—purely by luck, I'm sure—while my date won pretty much every other round.

Despite my less-than-stellar performance, the game was a blast. We had a lot of laughs and managed to get our steps in as we dashed from side to side, trying to retrieve the football. It's a fun and active way to spend a couple of hours.

Would I do this experience again? Probably. I did hurt

my back a couple of weeks before, so throwing footballs wasn't the most comfortable activity for me. But for $16 per person, you get access for as long as you want to play, which is a pretty good deal. Next time, I'd love to try the food there and bring along a group of friends for a lively game.

Tips if you want to try it:

- **Find a location:** If you're lucky enough to be near a Fowling Warehouse, definitely check it out. It's a unique and enjoyable night out.
- **Read the rules:** Brush up on the game rules beforehand to avoid any confusion during play.
- Stay hydrated: Bring a water bottle or buy one there—you'll need it after all that running around.

EXPERIENCE #20: SERVED UP SOME FUN PLAYING PICKLEBALL

Let me tell you about the latest fitness phenomenon sweeping the nation: pickleball. Yes, pickleball (not shocking!) To quote my new friend Lynn, whom I had the pleasure of meeting on this adventure, "Pickleball is like ping pong, only four times bigger, you put the table on the floor, stand up, and play." It's this fabulous mashup of ping pong, tennis and racquetball that's got everyone talking. Imagine ping pong decided to hit the gym, bulk up, and take its game outdoors.

So, how did I end up on a pickleball court? It all started with a Facebook invite from a guy named Paul (shoutout to Paul for making this happen). I'd heard of pickleball but never quite got around to trying it. When Paul suggested it, I figured, why not? Little did I know I was about to dive headfirst into one of the most entertaining sports out there.

When I walked into the local recreation center, I was greeted by a scene that looked like a cross between a pickleball tournament and a high-energy social gathering. The basketball courts had been transformed with removable tennis nets, and there were four games in full swing. It was like stepping into the heart of the pickleball universe.

To start, I placed my racket into a container, which felt oddly ceremonial—like I was relinquishing my hopes and dreams of being a pickleball prodigy. As games ended, my racket was shuffled along until it was my turn. Paul, who had been playing for almost a year, graciously lent me his racket for the day. I had no idea what I was doing, but I was ready to give it a shot.

The crowd was a delightful mix—lots of folks over 55, some teenagers, and a few midlifers. It was like a community mixer where everyone was bonding over their shared love of pickleball. And me? I was the newbie trying to figure out the rules while pretending I knew what I was doing.

When it was finally our turn on the court, Paul kindly informed our opponents that I was a complete rookie. As we played, Paul began giving me a crash course in pickleball. "Move up, go back, serve like this for better control." Soon, everyone on the court was chipping in with tips and tricks. It was like being adopted into a pickleball family, with everyone eager to help a first-timer like me. I learned about "the kitchen" (not where you find your coffee maker, but a no-volley zone), the double bounce rule (you've got to let the ball bounce once on each side before volleys), and that games can be played to

9 or 11 points, depending on how many people are waiting for their turn.

Despite my initial clumsiness, I started to get the hang of it. The game was much more dynamic than I expected, with a mix of strategy and agility. And the community? Absolutely fantastic. Everyone was so welcoming and supportive, making it a truly enjoyable experience.

Would I do this experience again? You bet! I'm definitely planning to get back on the court now that I've had a taste of what pickleball is all about. The game was a lot of fun, and the sense of community was heartwarming.

Tips if you want to try it:

- **Find Local Courts:** Look for pickleball courts in your area. Some places have dedicated pickleball facilities, while others use converted basketball courts.
- **Check Equipment Requirements:** See if you need to bring your own racket or if you can rent one on-site. Many places offer rentals.
- **Stay Hydrated:** Don't underestimate the workout! Bring a water bottle to keep hydrated, or buy one there.
- **Consider Lessons:** While not necessary, taking a lesson or two can be helpful, especially for first-timers. It can give you a solid foundation and save you from making some rookie mistakes.

- **Wear the Right Shoes:** Opt for shoes that provide good grip on a basketball court. You want to avoid slipping and sliding.
- **Protection Gear:** If you're prone to tennis elbow or knee issues, consider wearing some protective gear. It's better to be safe than sorry!

EXPERIENCE #21: GROOVED AT POLYPHONIC SPREE'S DEBUT SHOW AT THE DOME PLANETARIUM

A few months ago, I was having a casual conversation with a guy I was seeing at the time about taking a trip to Las Vegas. The main reason? To experience something truly out of this world—the newly built Sphere. If you haven't heard of it, The Sphere is the world's largest spherical structure designed for immersive visual and audio experiences. Not only can you watch mind-blowing programs on a massive 360-degree screen, but it also hosts concerts, merging live music with visuals for a fully immersive and epic experience. Honestly, it sounded divine. I was beyond excited, imagining how incredible it would be. But here's the twist—things didn't work out with the guy, and, as a result, neither did the trip to The Sphere. Oh well, so much for that.

Fast forward a few months, and I was scrolling through Facebook when an ad popped up for an event called *Atmosphere: The Ultimate Experience.* The name caught my eye, and it was being held at the University of

North Texas in their own planetarium dome—a much smaller version of The Sphere, but it sounded like a mini immersive experience I didn't want to miss. What really sealed the deal for me was the live music by *The Polyphonic Spree* accompanying the film. The promo video looked intriguing, even if it wasn't as grand as The Sphere, it had a cool, artsy vibe that was too good to pass up—plus, no plane tickets to Vegas were required.

I quickly convinced my two best guy friends, Craig and Andy, to get tickets, too. Andy and I decided to make an evening of it and headed to downtown Denton, TX, early to grab some good food before the show. Craig met us later, and we all set off together. **Side note**: universities offer such amazing opportunities! On our walk to the Planetarium, we saw a flyer advertising a study-abroad program to research penguins in Chile. How cool is that?! So, to all the younger readers of this book (yes, all two of you), take this middle-aged woman's advice: **seize every opportunity** that comes your way during college. Seriously, do it. Ok, mini-lecture over.

When we arrived at the Planetarium, it was much smaller than I expected, with maybe 70 seats. It wasn't packed, but the audience included a few actors from the film, which was kind of cool. The show's creator gave a brief introduction, explaining that the project was a labor of love years in the making. Musicians and designers from around the world had contributed, and it was clear this was his passion project—a dream brought to life.

The lights dimmed, and the show began with a peaceful scene of people sitting around a crackling campfire. Then, the camera zoomed into one person's eye, and suddenly, we were swept into a kaleidoscope of colors and shapes, accompanied by trippy, vibrant music. I couldn't help but smile—the whole thing felt like a wild, psychedelic ride. It actually reminded me of my one experience with mushrooms (which you can read about in Experience #28) where everything is amplified in your mind, and colors and sounds take on a life of their own. This felt the same, but minus the actual mushrooms.

The film shifted perspectives, diving into the lives of different characters, each told through a unique visual and audio style. Sometimes there was no real plot, just a dreamlike sequence of colors and sounds. Other times, there was a narrative, like one story about a man whose alcoholic father stole his guitar, leading him to follow a similar destructive path until, years later, he was gifted another guitar that changed his life. The vibrant visuals brought each scene to life in a way that was both mesmerizing and a little surreal.

There were a few moments where I had to close my eyes because the motion of the spinning visuals started to trigger some mild nausea. But after taking a breather, I was back into the flow of the experience, fully immersed in the wild display of art, music and storytelling.

After it ended, I asked Craig and Andy what they thought. Craig, who's always very analytical, said he wished the stories were more cohesive and had a stronger storyline. Andy, on the other hand, compared it to a tripped-out version of Disney's *Fantasia*, which I thought was a pretty accurate (and hilarious) description.

Personally, I enjoyed the show for what it was—an artistic, colorful escape that didn't require too much thinking. It was just the right length, too, clocking in at under an hour, which was enough to keep things interesting without dragging on.

There was one recurring theme that piqued my curiosity: a mysterious giant hand that appeared in several of the stories. After the show, I asked the creator about its meaning. He explained that the hand represented whatever higher power people believe in. It was open to interpretation— a good collegeiate answer. They even had a giant hand sculpture outside the Planetarium, tying it all together.

Would I do this again? I think so. I'm really glad I got to experience this mini-Sphere version close to home. If they put on a new show, I'd definitely be interested in going again.

Tips if you want to try it:

- Go with an open mind. You never know what you might experience.
- If you're prone to motion sickness, be prepared to close your eyes during the spinning visuals or sit near the back for less impact.
- If you're into psychedelics, this might be the perfect microdose experience without the actual substances (but to each their own).

EXPERIENCE #22: ENJOYED LIVE THEATER IN A VINTAGE RECORD STORE: LOVE AND VINYL

When my friend Greg, who lives in Oklahoma, asked me to do something, I said yes without a second thought. Greg and I have been friends for years, but it had been a solid seven years since we last hung out. Yes, seven! That's practically a lifetime in friend years. He drove down to Texas, and we caught up over dinner. We laughed so hard that I almost choked on my chicken, so when he suggested getting together again. I was all in. Greg promised to handle the details and find something fun for us to do, and let me tell you, he understood the assignment.

In the heart of East Dallas, there's this small but super nostalgic record store called Good Records. It's the kind of place that smells like vinyl and has the same cozy vibe as your grandma's attic—if your grandma was a hipster with a vibe for classic rock. The Kitchen Dog Theater Company decided to shake things up for their 33rd season by putting on plays in unconventional locations—

think Rough Riders Stadium, a CrossFit gym, a college campus, and yes, a record store. That's how we ended up at Good Records for a play called "Love and Vinyl."

Now, this play was written specifically for the record store setting, and they really made the most of it. Imagine chairs placed around giving us a super up-close-and-personal experience. It felt like we were all part of the cast —only we didn't have to memorize lines or wear costumes (thank goodness, because I had a hard enough time picking out an outfit for dinner). The play featured three characters: one guy who had just been dumped, his supportive friend, and the female record store owner.

As the story unfolded, the friend developed a serious crush on the store owner, but she wasn't exactly rolling out the red carpet for him. I mean, poor guy was trying to impress her while she was busy pricing vintage records and fixing a broken microwave. By the end of the play, though, they finally decided to leave the store and grab a drink together. It was a sweet, simple story that felt even more intimate because of the unique setting—like they were living out their own romantic comedy.

After the show, we were encouraged to browse the records in the store and maybe even buy one (because who can resist a good record?). Apparently, we could. We left empty-handed, my dreams of becoming the proud owner of a vintage vinyl collection dashed like my hopes of winning the lottery. But hey, sometimes the experience is worth more than the record, right? At least that's what I told myself as we walked back to the car, laughing about the night and wondering what other adventures awaited us—hopefully with fewer broken hearts and more albums next time!

Would I Do This Experience Again?

Absolutely! The idea of doing a play outside of a traditional theater and making the setting a part of the story was just brilliant. It made the experience feel fresh and unexpected—two things I'm always up for!

Tips if You Want to Try It:

- **Think Outside the Box:** If you're a theater lover, seek out performances in unconventional venues for a unique experience.
- **Embrace the Setting:** The setting can add so much to the story, so be open to plays in non-traditional spaces.
- **Suggest to Your Group:** If you're involved in theater, propose the idea of performing in a unique location. It could be a game-changer!
- **Explore After the Show:** Stick around after the play to explore the venue—whether it's a record store, a gym or a stadium. You never know what hidden gems you might find.

EXPERIENCE #23: EXPLORED THE WONDERS OF THE KENNEDY SPACE CENTER

Ah, Florida! The Sunshine State, home to sandy beaches, swampland and, of course, alligators. I ventured there to visit two of my friends from a previous job—Emma and Ila. Our grand plan was to kayak into the bioluminescent waters of Melbourne, a thrilling experience we were all eagerly anticipating. But as fate would have it, high winds canceled our kayak tour, and we were left scrambling for new adventures. We ziplined. We saw kangaroos out in the open, and we tasted gator. But there was something more we wanted to try, and strangely, it was a museum.

I usually don't get excited about museums. At. All. But the Kennedy Space Center? Think of it as a museum having a wild party with Disney. It was out of this world —pun very much intended! Emma had to head back to Jacksonville while Ila and I spent the last few hours together. She mentioned going to the Space Center, and I honestly had never thought about it. A museum? Bleh! Oh Staci of little Kennedy Space Center Faith.

We rolled up to the Kennedy Space Center around 1 p.m., buzzing with excitement. Not only was it a chance to explore space like never before, but we also hit the jackpot: a rocket launch was scheduled for that afternoon! Can you imagine our delight? Picture us like kids on a sugar high, but with slightly less sugar and more space geekery.

Our first stop was a vast room stuffed with space memorabilia. We're talking everything from historic rockets to moon-driving cars to actual spacesuits. It felt like wandering through a cosmic garage sale of epic proportions. We then made our way to the IMAX theater for a presentation called "Deep Space," which was all about the James Webb Telescope. And let me tell you, this thing cost $10 billion and took about 30 years to build.

Watching the film, I found myself in a teary-eyed state typically reserved for rom-coms. The scope of our universe and the miracle that the elements came together to allow us to exist was overwhelming. The James Webb Telescope is showing us sights we've never seen before, and some of them were absolutely breathtaking. One image, in particular, called Cosmic Cliffs, is essentially a star nursery seven light-years away. I was so moved by the miracle of space and honestly life on our planet, and what a miracle each one of us are to exist at all.

After drying some sentimental earthly tears, we hopped on the bus tour to check out the Apollo missions.

This was like stepping into a time machine that took us right into the heart of the Space Race. Learning about the brave souls who ventured into the unknown and the incredible missions they undertook was inspiring.

The Kennedy Space Center truly took my breath away —slow clap for space. Sadly, the rocket launch we were eagerly waiting for kept getting delayed until it was eventually called off. So, both the bioluminescence tour and the rocket launch were not quite as planned. But hey, we still made some stellar memories!

Would I do this experience again? Without a doubt! I can't wait to go back someday. I was genuinely in awe of the space discoveries and the incredible visuals. Plus, I got to see wild alligators from the tour bus—so win-win!

Tips if you want to try it:

- Plan for a full day. There's so much to see and do that you'll need the time.
- Bring water and snacks. Hydration and a little munchies can go a long way.
- Wear comfortable walking shoes. Trust me, your feet will thank you.
- If you're bringing kids and plan to catch one of the movies, sit on the exterior side for easy exits.
- Check out the app for rocket launches (Space Coast Launches). Rocket science, indeed!
- Look online for discounted tickets before you go. You might save a few bucks.

- Consider upgrading to the astronaut experience for an extra $30 if you're feeling extra adventurous.

EXPERIENCE #24: BECAME A GUEST ON A FAMOUS PODCAST

In August 2024, I posted the following on my Facebook page:

"I stalked myself tonight. I went back 7 years on my own FB page. Is that weird? (It's weird). I have dabbled back into the bizarre world of online dating, and I never feel good being back on the dating apps. If you've never used dating apps, it's like shopping for your next relationship on Amazon. You see a couple of pics, read the description, then order your person with delivery normally at a coffee shop. There are so many good people in this world, but you can totally lose sight of that on a dating app. I've met some great souls along the way, but y'all. It's exhausting.

I sometimes wonder, why am I single? Am I too picky? Am I a "meh" catch? Do I need to show more effort? Do I need to be more demure? So, I stalked myself. I went back almost 7 years. And you know what happened (tell us Staci what you found stalking yourself)? I was in tears at how grateful I am for my life! I saw my travels, family, friends, Zumba family, experiences, learning certificates, service... blessing after blessing after blessing. Although there have of course been some big challenges in my life, I've been sooooooo incredibly blessed to have lived my life to the fullest. Truly such a good reminder that what we focus on, expands. We can see the rose or the thorn. So, this is a little push to you ... stalk thyself! See all the goodness God/the universe/life has provided. PS... if you don't love what you see, it's never too late to start seeing the roses."

Yep. My dating and lack of partner lamentation ended quickly after being reminded again of what a blessing it is to be alive. Now, that doesn't mean I don't want a man to partner up with, but I also have let go of expectations of it happening. Imagine my surprise when just a few days later, the following mass email came to my inbox from Damona Hoffman:

"Hey there! Exciting news! After over two years, I'm bringing back live coaching on the Dates & Mates podcast, and this is your chance to get in on the action. You've probably seen me working my magic on the Drew Barrymore show as the Official Relationship Expert of that show. Now, it's your turn to get that same level of expert guidance! Take a peek at what my live coaching looks like on The Drew Barrymore Show!

Here's the scoop: I'm looking for two special individuals who are available for a recording session in the next two weeks. If you're feeling stuck in your dating life, I'm here to help you break through those barriers and find your path to love.

What's the catch? The only requirement is that you're willing to have your session recorded to air within The Dates & Mates Podcast and that you're available on a weekday between

9 a.m. - 6 p.m. PT to have the session with me sometime in the next week. Interested? Here's what to do: Reply to this email and share your story. Tell me why you want this coaching session and how you think it could change your dating life. Be open, be honest, and let your personality shine through! Don't miss this chance to get unstuck and kick-start your journey to finding love. Who knows what can happen? The last two people who did this with me found relationships within months and one of them just got married last fall.

Can't wait to hear from you! With love, Damona

P.S. Remember, I only have two spots available, so message me ASAP if you're interested! "

What do you think I did when I read that? If you guessed, you wrote something and sent it off, you win the prize! Here is what I wrote:

"Oh, my goodness! What a dream to be able to get a coaching session with you! I just finished your book a couple of weeks ago and it was gold!

I hope this message finds you surrounded by love and sanity —two things I seem to be running short on in the dating department!

I've just hit the big 5-0, and while I'm rocking the single life like a pro (cue Beyoncé's "Single Ladies"), I can't help but feel like something's missing. You see, I've had a wonderfully full life, but lately, online dating has turned into a never-ending loop of swiping, ghosting and enough small talk to fill a hundred first date. I feel icky now when I do online dating.

Remember the good old days when men actually planned first dates? Ah, nostalgia. Instead, I'm now the proud owner of a collection of "What's up?" messages that lead absolutely nowhere. I'm starting to wonder if I'm the one secretly sabotaging my love life. Could I be resisting potential matches? Or have I just had too many disappointing dates?

I'm reaching out because I need your help to break this cycle —or at least laugh about it along the way. Maybe it's time for me to shift my perspective, or perhaps I need to let go and let love happen (if it's out there somewhere between all those dating apps). I have deleted all of my apps and I would love to find love in the wild.

If you think you can handle the challenge that is my love life, I'd love to chat more and see if we're a match—strictly in the coaching sense, of course!

Thanks for considering my plea for help. I'm ready for some insight from the master.

Thanks,

Staci Berkovitz"

Guess what I got in my inbox? (I know, you read the title of this chapter, but let's at least pretend to be surprised). I made it through the first round ... then the second ... and finally the third! And just a few days after I sent my first email, I was selected to be on her podcast!

I know! What a great opportunity to get dating advice from a guru!

So, the day of the podcast recording (video and live), I curled my hair, put on make-up and nervously got ready for the virtual recording. Damona was as nice and real as can be both on and off camera. She asked me questions about my dating background and my online dating experience. While listening, she helped me dive deeper into what could potentially be blocking me. She also gave me ideas on how to meet people in real life, in addition to relearning how to flirt.

By the end of the hour, I felt inspired to accept the one-week flirt challenge as well as write a narrative about my person and how life will be with him in six months. Homework completed, although my flirting game needs major work.

Would I do this again? Oh boy! It was nerve-wracking. I have my own podcast but being on someone else's that has the listenership that she does, it made my armpits sweat. However, I did get so much out of the experience and was fortunate to meet such a wise person. So, the short answer is, yes.

Tips if you want to be a guest on a podcast:

- Know what it is you want to talk about.
- Make sure you have a good microphone, headset and camera.
- Life is short! Why not say yes!?!

EXPERIENCE #25: SAVORED A CULINARY ARTS DINING EXPERIENCE AT A COLLEGE

Ever had that moment when you're mindlessly scrolling through social media and someone posts a photo of food that looks so incredible, it makes your stomach grumble and your mouth water? You know the kind of food that screams, "You must have this right now, or you will regret it forever"? If you're nodding along, you're my kind of people. If not, I might need to question your taste buds— or at least your soul. Just kidding … sort of.

Anyway, this very scenario happened to me recently. A chef friend of mine shared a picture of some delectable seafood on Facebook, and I was instantly hooked. I had to find out where I could get my hands on that dish. Turns out, the local community college's culinary arts program was running a series of themed dining experiences as part of their final exams. For a modest fee, you could savor a meal prepared by the students themselves. This week's theme? Seafood.

Naturally, I dove straight into the link she provided,

only to find that all six available slots were already taken. Disappointment ensued. But, I wasn't ready to give up just yet. I signed up for the waiting list, crossing my fingers that someone would drop out.

A few weeks later, I got the coveted email saying a spot had opened up just in time for the next event. I immediately roped in my friend Carmon to join me. Carmon is a bit pickier with her food, so I wasn't entirely sure how thrilled she'd be about the Latin Caribbean themed menu that week. But hey, she's a trooper, so off we went.

We met at the campus's Red Room, the culinary dining space where the magic was to unfold. Outside the room, there were little gifts of veggie seeds encouraging visitors to plant their own gardens. I thought it was a charming touch—nothing says "farm-to-table" like growing your own ingredients!

We were seated promptly, and a student presented us with the special non-alcoholic drink of the night: a passion fruit mojito. It was... well, let's just say it was intensely sour. I stuck with water while Carmon bravely tried the drink, probably regretting it a bit.

The menu had been sent ahead, which was nice because it gave us a chance to ponder our choices. There were a few options for each course—appetizers, mains and desserts. The Latin Caribbean theme meant the menu was meat-heavy, which was a bit daunting but also intriguing.

For appetizers, we could choose between crispy cheese and cassava bites or a shrimp, pineapple and mango ceviche. We decided to try both, because why not? The cassava bites were the clear winner in my book—crunchy and delightful. For the main course, we had the choice of oxtail with beef wagyu tender, guava-glazed pork ribs or a Caribbean-style chicken sandwich with fries. We decided to be adventurous and went with the oxtail and pork ribs. We almost played it safe with the chicken sandwich, but where's the fun in that? Desserts included tres leches cake, flan or a donut. I was thrilled to see tres leches on the menu—always a yummy choice.

The food presentation was stunning—definitely worthy of a Facebook or Instagram post. The creativity was impressive, even if the flavors didn't always hit it out of the park. The wagyu beef and cassava bites were definitely highlights.

Overall, the experience was fantastic. It's amazing to see students getting hands-on experience in their field, and for just $15, it was a steal. We left with full bellies and big smiles, both impressed with the students' culinary talents and the value of the event.

Would I do this experience again? Absolutely! I'd love to try another themed dinner and now that I know about it, I'll be on the lookout for future events. Nothing beats good food, especially when it supports budding chefs.

Tips if you want to try it:

- Check out local community colleges or universities with culinary arts programs. They often have public dining events.
- Sign up early to avoid missing out.

- Prepare for some adventurous eating—it's all part of the fun!
- Bring your appetite and a sense of culinary adventure. And if you see a food photo that makes you drool, just remember: there's a whole world of delicious experiences out there waiting for you.

EXPERIENCE #26: EMBARKED ON A 24-HOUR PHONE FAST AND SURVIVED

My name is Staci, and I'm about to confess something that might sound all too familiar: I'm hopelessly addicted to my phone. If you're nodding in agreement, you're definitely not alone. If not, well, you might just be a mystical being from another planet. Joking aside, the allure of social media and constant notifications can be incredibly compelling.

A few months ago, I read "How to Break Up with Your Phone" by Catherine Price. This book was like a wake-up call with a side of tough love. It explored why we're all so distracted and suggested a radical idea: a 24-hour phone fast. I knew I had to try it, though finding the perfect 24-hour window felt as challenging as winning the lottery. Between work, family and a thousand daily commitments, it seemed impossible to carve out a whole day without my phone.

But in March 2024, I finally decided to dive in

headfirst. I picked a Friday night at 9:30 PM to Saturday night at 9:30 PM for my phone detox. My schedule was simple: teach a Zumba class and hit the grocery store. I made a pact with myself—my phone would come along (turned off) just for emergencies and then be recharged once I got home. I was ready for a day of disconnection.

The first hurdle came in the middle of the night. As a middle-aged woman, frequent bathroom trips are just part of the routine. But what wasn't routine was my automatic reach for my phone. I had it stashed across the room, so I couldn't get it, but wow, what a habit I'd formed! It felt like trying to break a sleepwalking routine —awkward and slightly disorienting.

The next morning, I gave myself a little extra sleep before heading out to teach Zumba. I let my students know about my phone-free day, which meant no filming or snapping pictures of our energetic class. Just as we were getting into the rhythm, my trusty iPod (yes, I still use one—vintage, I know) decided to quit on me. Cue the existential crisis! My Spotify playlist, which I'd planned to use for the class, was on my phone. With over 50 people waiting for their Zumba fix, I had to make a tough call. I turned on my phone, pulled up Spotify, and played the music. After the class, I asked one of my students to turn the phone off for me. It felt like a small but significant victory in my phone-free quest.

After Zumba, I ventured to the grocery store (phone out of sight) and then returned home for a day of leisurely productivity. I tackled meal prep for the week.

The rest of the day unfolded with a satisfying mix of laundry, vacuuming my car and indulging in a luxurious bath while reading a book. I read more outside the bath and then journaled, I rounded off the day with some yoga and reflection, and before I knew it, my 24 hours were up.

When I finally turned my phone back on, I recorded a fresh podcast episode, still buzzing from my phone-free experience. Then, I tackled my Duolingo Spanish lessons, feeling a sense of accomplishment. I had 46 unread messages waiting for me, but they seemed almost quaint after a day of unplugged serenity. I realized how much more peaceful I felt without my phone constantly demanding my attention.

Would I do this experience again? Without a doubt. I'd love to make it a regular part of my routine, maybe once a month. It was a fantastic reset, offering a clear perspective on how tethered I am to my phone and how liberating it can be to disconnect.

Tips if you want to try it:

- Choose a 24-hour period when you don't need to leave your home. This makes it easier to stay off your phone and avoids the temptation of using it out of necessity.
- Prepare with engaging alternatives. Have books, games, puzzles or other activities ready to keep yourself occupied and entertained.
- Inform your regular contacts about your phone fast. Let them know you'll be unreachable for

the next 24 hours, especially those who might worry if they don't hear from you.

- Make a list of urgent tasks. Note anything you need to handle on your phone so you can let go of the anxiety about what you might be missing.

EXPERIENCE #27: POOPED WITH COLOGUARD FOR A COLONOSCOPY

Ah, the joys of turning 50! With it comes a rite of passage that's less about celebratory cake and more about ... poop. Yep, I'm talking about a colonoscopy. If you're like me, the thought of colon prep sounds delightful, right? Let's be honest, it's not exactly a topic that gets the party started.

At 50, or even 45 according to the latest recommendations, it was time to tackle this preventative procedure head-on (or butt on). It's one of those necessary evils if you want to stay on top of your health. To make matters more real, I was recently at a dinner celebrating my friend's bachelorhood when my phone lit up with a call from another friend detailing her epic colonoscopy prep ordeal. It was the kind of conversation that makes you want to curl up and hide. My bachelor friend, in the midst of wedding festivities, nonchalantly mentioned he uses Cologuard instead. It sounded so much like a commercial I half-expected him to start listing side effects.

Cologuard is a home testing kit that lets you do your own screening from the comfort of your bathroom. It's a bit like the VIP lounge of colonoscopies. You order the kit online, and your insurance will often cover it since it's a preventative measure. The process starts with a quick online questionnaire to see if Cologuard is suitable for you or if you'd be better off with the traditional in-person screening. Given my risk factors, I was all set for the at-home adventure.

Once approved, you can opt for a free call from a doctor to go over any questions. I decided to take advantage of this, if only to have someone explain the finer points of the process. The call was brief but helpful, emphasizing the importance of reading the instructions carefully.

The big day arrived, and it was time for the grand poop event. The kit included a container, some liquid and a comprehensive instruction manual that felt like it could double as a novella. The process involved placing a collection device under your toilet seat, doing your business, and then transferring a sample into the provided container. As for delivery, I chose home pickup —there was no way I was strutting into UPS with my sample in hand.

Within less than 10 days, I received the results. All clear! It was a relief, and I felt like I'd conquered a personal milestone.

Would I do this again? Well, let's just say I'm not signing up for a weekly version of this experience, but I would definitely opt for Cologuard again for the sake of prevention. It's a handy option for those who prefer to avoid the traditional prep and have a bit more control over their schedule. Just check with your insurance to understand how frequently they cover the test—whether it's yearly, every five years or whatever your plan dictates.

Tips if you want to try it:

- **Check Eligibility:** Make sure you meet the criteria for Cologuard by completing the online questionnaire. It will determine if this at-home test is suitable for you or if a traditional colonoscopy is needed.
- **Review Instructions:** Once you receive your kit, carefully read the instructions. It's crucial to follow them exactly to ensure accurate results.
- **Plan for Privacy:** The process involves collecting a sample, so ensure you have privacy and enough time to complete it without interruptions.
- **Choose Home Pickup:** If you're not keen on delivering your sample in person, opt for the home pickup service to save yourself some stress (and not having to take your poop to the post office).
- **Check Insurance Coverage:** Confirm with your insurance how often they cover Cologuard and any other preventative screenings. Coverage can vary, so it's good to know what to expect.

- **Stay Informed:** If you have any questions or uncertainties, utilize the free doctor call that comes with the kit. It's a great way to get clarification and peace of mind.
- **Keep a Positive Attitude:** It's a necessary step for health, so approach it with a sense of humor and positivity. After all, it's all about keeping things in check!

EXPERIENCE #28: GOT GROOVY AND EMBRACED THE VIBES WITH MUSHROOMS

I think I need to preface this chapter by saying that I'm not a drinker or drug user. I can count on two hands how many times I've had a drink in my life, and I've never been drunk. I wear that with a bit of a badge of honor because, over the years, I've learned more about alcohol and seen how it can lead people down some pretty questionable paths. So, staying away feels like a win. The only drug I've ever tried is weed. My high school girlfriends and I once tried to score the rolled kind during a Girls Trip to Colorado, but let's just say our attempt was more comedy than success. Despite the bag of Doritos and searching YouTube for tips, we failed. I tried the chewable version three times: once with a boyfriend who was, in hindsight, not the best person to experiment with (he was rather unstable), and twice more for sleep, which left me with a monster headache. My weed phase was brief, to say the least. I also had a forgettable encounter with Ayahuasca at a church in Texas, which was more "meh" than memorable. So, when my close friend (let's call her E) offered to guide me through a mushroom experience, I was hesitant. She had raved about the profound transformations she and her boyfriend had experienced, assuring me that mushrooms could be a powerful source of healing.

Let's talk about mushrooms (and no, not the Portobello kind you throw on a grill). For those unfamiliar, mushrooms, or shrooms, are also known as psilocybin. According to *ScienceAlert*, these mushrooms can cause hallucinations, pupil dilation and other effects. They are increasingly being studied for their potential benefits in treating anxiety and trauma. Sounds like a trip, right? Pun intended.

She reassured me that her experiences with mushrooms had been deeply spiritual and promised to make sure the setting was safe and uplifting. So, on the day of my shroom adventure, we went to her church and enjoyed a heartfelt message about mothers (it was Mother's Day weekend). Feeling all the feels, we headed back to her apartment to walk the dogs and discuss what to expect. When we returned, she had me write a letter to my future self, 10 years from now and list the areas of growth I wanted to focus on. I also created a playlist of uplifting music to accompany the experience. Then, it was showtime.

"E" asked if I wanted a breakthrough or just an experience, which would determine the dosage. I said I wanted an experience but was open to a breakthrough if it happened. With that information, she measured out the dosage—3 grams for me and 1 gram for her—and made a tea with hot water and lemon. We let it steep for 15 minutes, and then it was time to drink up.

The effects hit "E "first, but it took a little longer for me. When I looked at her, I saw her morphing between an old woman and a young woman, like some sort of magical time traveler. She spoke to me about my mom and her love for me, and also about her own grandfather and how much he needed love. Every time I closed my eyes, I saw eyes—kind, friendly eyes that looked like they belonged in a Pixar film. We spent a lot of time in silence, soaking in the music I had chosen. Then "E" asked me to talk about my dating life.

I explained that earlier that day, I had gone on a date at a casual dining place. When I arrived at the restaurant for the date, the guy was already sitting there with his meal. "E" looked at me, appalled, and said, "No more! Enough dating guys who aren't kings. No more wasting time with men who aren't at your level. No more dating guys who aren't ready. You journal every day about what you want, but you're not dating to those expectations. You're almost 50. It's time to date kings. Remember, the universe is watching!"

I was taken aback. I hadn't mentioned that I'd been seeing eyes the whole time, but her words made the connection clear: The universe is watching, and it was time to focus on dating "kings."

The high from the mushrooms lasted about four hours and was a beautiful spiritual experience. E's boyfriend had made a delicious Aryuvedic vegan soup for afterward. By the time it was almost midnight, I was exhausted. I went into the bathroom to get ready for bed and looked in the mirror. I looked like I had just walked off the set of a sci-fi movie—my eyes appeared unusually large due to the lingering effects. If I'd seen myself in that moment, I might have thought I was auditioning for the role of "Extra from Another Planet."

Would I do this experience again? Possibly. I'm glad I tried it, though I'm not sure if it's something I'd do frequently or just remember it as a one-time event.

Tips if you want to try it:

- **Ensure a Safe Environment:** Make sure you're in a safe, comfortable place with people you trust completely. A supportive setting is crucial. It's not the time to be in a crowded café or a random party.
- **Avoid Mirrors:** It's easy to get distracted or unsettled by your own reflection, so it's best to avoid looking in mirrors. Trust me, seeing your own eyes staring back at you in a psychedelic state can be unsettling.
- **Stick to Uplifting Content:** Don't watch anything scary or listen to anything that might be unsettling. Opt for music or content that is positive and calming. No horror movies or breakup ballads!
- **Understand Individual Variability:** Everyone's experience can be different. Some might have profound, healing revelations, while others

may encounter overwhelming emotions. Be prepared for a range of outcomes and have a sense of humor about it.

- **Talk to Your Guides:** If you have any concerns or questions, communicate openly with your guides or facilitators. They can help navigate the experience and provide support. Think of them as your shroom sherpas.
- **Know the Risks:** Psychedelic experiences can be intense and may bring up unexpected emotions or insights. Approach them with an open mind, but be aware of the potential for challenging moments.
- **Reflect Afterwards:** Give yourself time to process the experience and reflect on any insights gained. Journaling or talking with a trusted friend can help integrate the experience into your daily life. Plus, it's a great way to document how you felt like an intergalactic explorer for a few hours.

EXPERIENCE #29: SAILED AWAY AT WHITE ROCK LAKE

Dating apps can be a wild ride. For those who haven't experienced the swipe-left/swipe-right phenomenon, picture shopping in a giant catalog—tons of options, but none seem quite right. Sometimes, you find a gem, and sometimes, it's like shopping for socks at a clearance sale. But every now and then, you hit the jackpot. Like the time I went sailing on White Rock Lake.

I matched with someone on Bumble, and instead of the usual coffee or drinks (which, let's face it, are as exciting as watching paint dry), I was in the "HAVE FUN ERA." If I was going to go on a date, it had to be something I'd enjoy, no matter who I was with. Enter Popeye—yes, that's what I'll call him. He was a sailing enthusiast, had his own sailboat, and was raised on the water. So, I suggested sailing. Why not, right?

White Rock Lake is a reservoir in Dallas, not a real lake, according to local lore. The story goes that it was once a tree-lined valley where Native Americans hunted bison. Fast forward to the early 1900s, and voila—White Rock Lake was born to help with the city's water shortage. The lake has a bit of a checkered history, including work by prisoners of war and a reputation for occasional mysterious happenings. So naturally, it was a prime spot for a first date.

On a beautiful May evening, I met Popeye at the boathouse. There was a birthday party in full swing, so the boathouse was buzzing with activity. Popeye had the boat ready, but before we could set sail, he had to use the boathouse's emergency boat to assist a stranded kayaker. That was my first clue that I was in good hands.

We set out on the lake, and Popeye gave me a crash course in sailing. I was tasked with hooking and releasing the sail—basically, if you don't duck, you get hit by the sail. For a couple of hours, we sailed, laughed and enjoyed the sunset. I also played duck or get hit" for most of the two hours. It was an entertaining, serene and picturesque experience.

After we returned, we walked around the boathouse and checked out the spider-webbed boats (apparently a hot spot for eight-legged friends). We said our goodbyes, and while there was no romantic spark, we both enjoyed the evening. He wasn't my forever Popeye, and I wasn't his Olive Oyl.

Would I do this again? Absolutely. It was a charming experience, and I'd love to try sailing on a bigger boat someday.

Tips if you want to try sailing:

- **Pick a good time:** Go for a beautiful evening when the weather is pleasant but be prepared for mosquitoes.
- **Be open to learning:** Get ready for a quick lesson on sailing—embrace it and remember to duck!
- **Safety first:** Make sure you're with someone who knows what they're doing and check the local history for any quirks about the location.

EXPERIENCE #30: TRIED A WHOLE FOODS PLANT-BASED DIET

As a health and wellness coach, I'm always preaching about cutting down on processed foods. I manage to follow this advice about 70% of the time. But let's be honest—if a bag of Cheetos lands in front of me, I'm all in. No shame, just Cheetos dust and a moment of pure, crispy bliss. So, I decided it was time for a real challenge: a whole foods plant-based diet for a week. My curiosity was piqued by a friend who had managed to cure her debilitating arthritis with this diet, and I wanted to see what it could do for me.

Lucky for me, my friend Tana was hosting a Whole Foods Plant-Based Diet info night at her house. For just $15, I could learn all about this eating style and sample some of the dishes. Clearly, this was an opportunity I couldn't pass up!

When I walked into her house, I was greeted by a PowerPoint presentation and a formidable stack of reference books. The first book on top was a vehement anti-cheese documentary (okay, maybe a slight exaggeration), so I braced myself for some intense, cheese-free enthusiasm.

Her presentation was fantastic. She shared her healing journey, the science behind the diet and the practicalities of incorporating whole foods into everyday life. Then came the part I was most excited about—the cooking demo. First on the menu was her green smoothie, which she made using fresh mint from her garden. She explained the ingredients: mint, spinach, frozen bananas, flax and chia seeds and water. It was a refreshing green concoction that tasted way better than it looked. The best part? She taught us how to store it in mason jars for a few days, which was a game-changer for meal prep.

Next up were chocolate chip cookies. These weren't your average cookies; they were sweetened with dates, and they contained no eggs, no regular flour and no butter. I had five. Yes, five. They were that good. She also made pancakes and a tofu egg scramble, both of which were unexpectedly delicious. I even tried to persuade her to come home with me and cook for me every day, leaving her five kids and husband behind. As of this writing, she has not taken me up on that offer.

The evening was so inspiring that I decided to give the whole foods plant-based diet a serious shot for five days. I was determined to go all in, so I turned to ChatGPT to create a meal plan, recipes and a grocery list. Sunday was dedicated to prepping all my meals for the week. This included smoothies, black bean and corn salad, hummus with veggies, and overnight oats. I also attempted to bake cookies with mashed bananas, applesauce, oats and dark chocolate chips—let's just say they were an acquired taste.

Dining out posed a challenge. With no flours, sugars, animal proteins, dairy or oils, finding suitable options at restaurants like Flower Child and Cava was tricky. While I managed to make it work, the experience was far from the culinary indulgences I'm used to.

Would I do it again? Absolutely. But with some adjustments. By the end of the five days, I felt a bit hungry and low on energy, especially during my fitness classes. If I were to try this again, I'd incorporate sweet or regular potatoes for added calories, include protein shakes and maybe add some tuna, eggs and olive oil to create a more balanced, sustainable diet.

Tips if you want to try it:

- **Listen to Your Body:** Monitor how you feel throughout the week. If you're constantly hungry or low on energy, it's a sign to adjust your intake.
- **Clear Out Temptations:** Get rid of any processed snacks and sweets from your house before starting. Cravings can be intense, and it's easier to stick to the diet if you don't have temptations within reach.
- **Prep and Plan:** Thoroughly prep your meals and snacks ahead of time. Having protein-rich

options and healthy snacks readily available will keep you on track and prevent you from reaching for less healthy alternatives.

EXPERIENCE #31: FLEW ON A PRIVATE JET TO STEAMBOAT SPRINGS, COLORADO

For most of my birthdays, I've been known to hunker down and brace for impact. My 30s and early 40s were not exactly birthday bonanzas, so I shifted gears in my late 40s to celebrate in more enjoyable ways—think lunches, dinners and small gatherings. When I turned 50, a friend planned a surprise party (which turned out to be a delightful, friend-filled celebration) a few days after my actual birthday. So, on the day of my birthday (a Thursday), I found myself without plans. To top it off, the Dallas Fort Worth area was hit by a hurricane-like storm, with winds so fierce they knocked out power and downed decades old trees. We were in the dark—literally and figuratively—for five days, with one of those days falling on my birthday. Faced with the prospect of spending the night without A/C, I decided to check into a hotel.

But hang tight, because this story takes a surprisingly

delightful turn. I had been seeing a guy who had mentioned that he owned a private jet due to his business travel commitments. He had casually offered, "If you ever want to go on a trip, just let me know." Well, with a new job starting the week after my birthday, I realized it was now or never. He was all in as well. So, we planned a day trip to Steamboat Springs, Colorado, to go hiking. And yes, we would be flying there on his private jet (cue hair flip and imaginary Prada bag).

On the morning of my birthday, I checked out of the hotel and drove to his place. He greeted me with a smoothie (extra points for that!), and we headed to the nearby airport—just a 10-minute drive. Get ready for this: We drove directly onto the tarmac beside the plane, where the airport staff awaited us. They took our luggage, loaded it onto the jet, and even parked our car for us. We had to walk only 15 steps from the car to the plane. No TSA lines, no crowds—just seamless, luxury travel. It was the ultimate way to start my 50th birthday.

As we boarded the jet, I marveled at the interior. The jet had six seats, including those for the pilot and co-pilot. There was a small mini-bar and a compact bathroom. The leather seats could be adjusted to be closer or farther from the person next to you, and while the cabin wasn't exactly tall enough for standing, you could still maneuver by crouching.

The flight was swift, effortless and an absolute blast!

After the luxurious jet ride, you knew we had to land somewhere equally as spectacular. Enter Steamboat

Springs. My 50th birthday kicked off with a flight fit for a rock star and landed in this charming mountain town, which turned out to be as picturesque as a postcard. It was summer, and the town was awash in greenery, wildflowers gracing the mountainsides like nature's confetti. Although Steamboat Springs is celebrated as a winter ski haven, experiencing it in the summer was nothing short of magical.

With only a day and a half to savor the beauty of Steamboat Springs, we knew we had to maximize every moment. Our adventure began at the local grocery store, where we assembled a culinary masterpiece for our hike: sushi, fruit, Cheetos, Doritos, and nut mixes. A lunch of champions, indeed. I struck up conversations with locals and did some quick Googling to pinpoint the best spots. We decided to conquer the Emerald Lake Trail.

Emerald Lake Trail was as enchanting as it sounds. The hike was a feast for the eyes, with every step offering new vistas of lush landscapes and wildflower-dotted slopes. When we reached the summit, my hiking companion—let's call him the "Jet Guy"—pulled out a rock for me to sit on and set up a picnic. The view was so breathtaking that it felt like a scene from a movie. As we relaxed, taking in the panoramic beauty, I couldn't help but feel a profound sense of gratitude.

As we began our descent, the adventure took an exciting turn. We spotted a bear—majestic, enormous and surprisingly close! The sighting was thrilling but not alarming; we managed to keep a respectful distance while we followed the bear's leisurely stroll through the neighborhood. The experience felt like a scene straight out of a nature documentary, and we were giddy!

Post-hike, we checked into our gorgeous hotel with breathtaking views of the mountain. True to my preference, we had separate rooms (a lady must maintain her standards, after all). We then explored downtown Steamboat Springs, a place brimming with charm. The town offered a perfect blend of touristy fun and genuine local vibe. Dinner was at Aura, a delightful spot nestled next to a rushing river. The nachos were divine—nachos on your birthday should be a universally accepted tradition! We finished the day unwinding in the hot tub, where we soaked our tired muscles while gazing at the majestic mountain views. It was the perfect end to an unforgettable day.

The next morning, we set off on another hike, this time tackling the Spring Creek Trail. Conveniently located near our resort, this trail offered a different kind of natural splendor, with waterfalls cascading and rivers flowing alongside our path. The serene environment made it an ideal hike, offering both beauty and tranquility. After our hike, we relaxed at a cozy sports bar for lunch next to a river, enjoying a laid-back meal that perfectly complemented the day's adventures.

Steamboat Springs turned out to be the ideal birthday destination, combining natural beauty with outdoor excitement. The trip was everything I had hoped for and more, and I'd definitely return to explore even further (even if I am not arriving by jet).

Would I do this again? Is the sky blue? Do Cheetos taste amazing? Is Arizona sweltering in the summer? Absolutely, yes! Sign me up for a repeat performance anytime for both the jet and Steamboat Springs.

Tips if you want to try it:

- **Jump at the Chance:** If you ever get the opportunity to fly on a private jet, seize it! It's an incredibly unique and luxurious way to travel that you'll remember fondly.
- **Embrace the Convenience:** Enjoy the no-fuss travel experience—no long lines, no security hassles, just smooth sailing (or flying, in this case).
- **Prepare for Spoiling:** Be ready to be pampered —private jets often come with amenities that make travel feel like a true VIP experience.
- **Timing is Everything:** While Steamboat Springs is renowned for its winter skiing, the late spring or early summer offers a different kind of charm. The weather is perfect, and you'll avoid the peak tourist season, making for a more serene experience.
- **Hike Smart:** The AllTrails app is your best friend for discovering the most scenic hikes in the area. From serene lakes to cascading waterfalls, the trails cater to all levels of hiking enthusiasts.
- **Plan for a Stay:** To fully embrace all that Steamboat Springs has to offer, plan for at least

three days. This will give you ample time to enjoy multiple hikes, savor local cuisine and soak in the town's picturesque ambiance.

UNTITLED

Experience #32: Partied at a Bingo Rave and Won Big

EXPERIENCE #32:
CELEBRATED AT A
TRADITIONAL MAYON
SHOWER

I've always had a soft spot for exploring different cultures. For years, I dreamt of attending an Indian wedding—dancing, vibrant music, stunning outfits, and let's not forget the samosas! A few years ago, a friend's daughter got married and invited me to the wedding. It was everything I imagined: a short, sweet ceremony followed by dancing that made my feet beg for mercy. It was perfect.

So, when one of my Zumba students, Humera, told me about her daughter's upcoming nuptials and invited me to the bridal shower, I was a strong, immediate yes! The family is from Pakistan, and in their culture, the bridal shower is called a Mayon. This event is traditionally held a few days before the wedding, where the bride is pampered, celebrated, and relieved of any responsibilities (she's not supposed to lift a finger between the Mayon and the wedding). Where can I sign up for that plan?

My fellow Zumba instructor and friend, Amanda, was also invited. Humera made sure we had the date marked on our calendars and even arranged for outfits to be sent from Pakistan for us to wear. When they arrived, I was floored. My outfit was an orange and gold top paired with a colorful, sequined skirt. I felt like royalty—move over, Cinderella, there's a new princess in town Pakistani style!

The invitation said the party would start at 6 p.m., so Amanda and I decided to meet at 5:30 and go together. But on the day of the event, we got a message from Humera: "Don't come until 7 p.m." Apparently, fashionably late is not just a suggestion—it's a mandate.

It was July of 2024, and as you can imagine, it was scorching hot in Texas. While the outfits were gorgeous, they were not designed for the blazing Texas heat. On our way there, I unceremoniously hiked up my skirt to cool off, apologizing to Amanda for the less-than-princess-like behavior. When we arrived, we were among the first to show up—so much for being cool by arriving late. The real cool cats (a term that I can use now that I am 50) strolled in even later. The room began to fill with women of all ages, all dressed in stunning outfits. A yellow and pink flower backdrop was set up for the bride, and all the family members wore yellow. I later learned that the yellow is traditional because turmeric is used in the ceremony, and if it stains their clothes, at least it blends in. Beautiful and practical—how can you not love that?

Someone started playing a drum, and before we knew it, the room was filled with singing. We were all melting a bit since the A/C wasn't on, but it added to the authenticity of the experience—it felt like we were actually outside in Pakistan in the middle of summer.

The bride finally made her grand entrance at 9 p.m., escorted under a tent-like structure (a scarf held by family and friends). She sat on the seat with the beautiful backdrop, and the feeding ceremony began. She was given sweet treats and money—an interesting twist that I later found out goes to charity. They also applied a turmeric paste to her, which I learned is part of the traditional rituals.

After what felt like a million pictures, we were invited to eat. At this point, we were sweaty and starving, so we eagerly filled our plates with delicious traditional food. I wasn't expecting the spice to be so spicy, but it was still mouth-wateringly good.

As the night wound down, we said our goodbyes to the bride and made our way out. Since shoes weren't allowed in the house, there were about 70 pairs scattered outside. Amanda didn't realize it at the time, but when she got home, she discovered that her sandals were intertwined with someone else's shoelaces. All is fair in love and Mayon, I suppose.

Would I do this experience again? Absolutely! Any chance to don these beautiful outfits is a yes! But next time, I'm hoping for a cooler month.

Tips if you want to try it:

- Do some reading beforehand: When I initially got the invite, I thought it was for the wedding.

I only found out it was a bridal shower when I decided to do some last-minute research on the day of the event. Having some background information definitely helped me appreciate the experience even more.

- Prepare for the heat: If you're attending a summer Mayon, be ready to sweat it out— especially if the A/C decides to take a day off.
- Embrace the fashionably late arrival: Seriously, showing up late is not just a good idea—it's practically required.

EXPERIENCE #33: PLANTED A VEGETABLE GARDEN

I kill things. There, I said it. You must know this about me. These poor, innocent things just want a chance to live the measure of their creation. But it doesn't matter—they are goners in my hands. What am I speaking about? Anything plant, grass, veggie or fruit-related. If it's green and growing, it's on death row with me.

I've tried to plant things—you know, to live off the land like our ancestors did. Let me tell you, if I had to rely on my gardening skills for survival, I'd be the star of my own tragic, one-episode reality show called *Starved in Seven Days*. But I was determined to have my own set of food one day, especially after witnessing the pure joy on my granddaughter's face when she saw her basil shoot sprout in a cup. That little green sprout brought her so much happiness, and I thought, "Why not me?" Plus, I watched a friend casually clip some mint from her garden to toss into her smoothie like it was no big deal. I was in awe. It was time to get my green thumb on.

So off I went to a local nursery/farm feed store, and for good measure, I hit up Home Depot too. I was all in. I decided on the following: tomatoes, red peppers, basil, oregano, spearmint and a lemon tree—because why not aim high? I also picked up two citronella plants to help with the ever-present mosquito population, because if I was going to be out there watering my mini-farm, I wasn't about to donate blood to the local insect life.

A friend of mine came over to help me plant the goods, and I made a solemn pledge to keep these plants alive, even if the hot Texas sun tried to steal my joy. We had a week of heavy rain, which gave my little garden the kickstart it needed. Before I knew it, the green tomatoes that had appeared on the plants turned red and were ready to eat. I clipped some basil, threw it in a dish and had my very own Italian feast. Okay, maybe calling it a feast is a stretch, but humor me, y'all—I grew it myself!

Fast forward to the middle of summer. The spearmint didn't make it. Despite my best efforts with watering, it dried up within a couple of weeks. The oregano gave me a taste of its potential before it too met its untimely demise. The basil, though, thrived wonderfully (and I learned you have to cut the flowers off right away, or the plant will stop growing—who knew?). The red pepper plant grew tall and proud ... but didn't produce a single pepper. The lemon tree? Well, its leaves became a gourmet meal for a very hungry grasshopper. But the tomatoes, oh, the tomatoes—they grew! I'm officially part of the Green Thumb Crew. T-shirts are being made as we speak.

Would I do this experience again? I think so. I'm a wiser gardener now and realize that there are things that can be done for better results (like, hello, Miracle-Gro). If I decide to plant another garden next spring, I'll start early and do some actual research on the best ways to care for them. Who knows? Maybe next time, I'll get a pepper or two.

Tips if you want to try it:

- **Water Daily:** Make sure you have time to water your plants every day; neglecting this is a fast track to failure.
- **Grow What You Eat:** Choose plants that you'll actually enjoy eating—no point in growing something you won't touch.
- **Start Small:** Begin with one or two types of plants to see how it goes before committing to a full-on garden.
- **Research Helps:** Learn the best ways to care for your chosen plants—Miracle-Gro and a little research can make a big difference.

UNTITLED

Experience #34: Ventured into Tantra Dating and
Embraced New Connections

EXPERIENCE #35: BECAME A NEBRASKA HUSKER FOR A DAY

In 2020, I accomplished one of my life goals: visiting all 50 states in the United States. Three states, however, barely got more than a friendly drive-through—Ohio, Kansas, and Nebraska. Kansas has since redeemed itself with two visits to see my son and his wife. Ohio is still on the deeper-dive list, especially for a proper fall exploration. That left Nebraska—yet to get the attention it deserved.

Earlier in the year, my friend Rachel and I took advantage of a sweet deal from Southwest Airlines: buy two tickets, and one of us would fly free in September. We were excited! However, by the time we got around to planning, our options were limited unless we wanted to spend the majority of the weekend in airports or on planes. After some searching, we landed on an unexpected destination: Omaha, Nebraska. Yes, Omaha!

When I started Googling things to do in Omaha, the one place that consistently popped up was the Omaha Henry Doorly Zoo and Aquarium, touted as the #1 zoo in the nation. Naturally, it became priority number one on our list. As for the rest of our weekend, we'd figure it out on the fly.

A few days before the trip, I had a sudden urge to experience the real heart of Nebraska—Husker football. What better way to do that than by going to a game at the University of Nebraska? Little did I know, securing tickets for a Huskers game isn't for the faint of heart. They've sold out every game since 1962—399 consecutive sellouts. After an exhausting search through resale websites, I finally scored two tickets. Go Big Red!

The day of our trip arrived, but it didn't start off smoothly. Our flight was delayed by over two hours, cutting into our precious weekend time. Nevertheless, we were determined to make the most of it. Once we landed, we hopped into our rental car and headed straight for downtown Omaha. To our surprise, it was charming! The rooftops were lush with plants and flowers, and the Old Market Passageway was a hidden gem—an alleyway between two buildings overflowing with greenery.

Rachel, being the shopping enthusiast that she is, dragged me into several shops, including one that sold the cutest (and best-smelling) soap. Then we stumbled upon Hollywood Candy, a massive retro candy store that transported me straight back to childhood. Candy cigarettes, rock candy, every Pez flavor and container imaginable—it was all there. And it didn't stop at candy; they had rooms full of pinball machines, vintage arcade games, records, and even life-sized cutouts of Hollywood stars. It was like a mashup of Willy Wonka's factory,

Hollywood nostalgia, and my childhood hangout, Spencer's. We didn't buy any candy, but we spent ages wandering through this quirky wonderland.

After a full day of traveling and exploring, we were exhausted and ready to rest up for the big game. We checked into our Airbnb, which turned out to be a room in a stunning old mansion across from the Joslyn Castle. Yes, Omaha has a castle! Built in the 1880s, it was an architectural marvel, and the grounds were perfect for a relaxing walk (which we didn't quite get to).

Game day arrived, and we headed to Lincoln, about an hour's drive from Omaha, to grab a bite at a place called Lazlo's before the game. Finding parking was a feat in itself with all the tailgaters around, so we ended up walking about ten blocks to the restaurant. There we met Ben, the world's friendliest waiter and a college student who gave us a crash course on all things Nebraska. Fun fact: with just two major cities—Omaha and Lincoln—80% of the state is rural farmland. During game days, the stadium becomes the second most populated "city" in the state. Ben also introduced us to the concept of "Nebraska Nice," a term that perfectly describes the locals' warm and welcoming nature.

At the stadium, I was blown away by the sea of red. The stands were filled with thousands of devoted fans, all decked out in the Huskers' signature color, creating a truly electric atmosphere. Even when the referees made a questionable call, the guy behind us remained polite—Nebraska Nice, indeed. One of the coolest moments was after the third quarter, when everyone turned on their phone flashlights, and the stadium lights went dark for a breathtaking light show. On windier nights, they even add a drone show, but alas, the wind wasn't in our favor that day.

After the light show, we decided to beat the traffic and left early, but not before running into one of my best friends who was there watching her son play. After a quick hug, we faced the long trek back to our car—over a mile away in a distant parking lot in Husker Land.

The next morning, we fueled up at a cheekily named breakfast spot called "Good Lookin'" before heading to the Omaha Zoo. The zoo offers two ticket options: the basic package, which includes the zoo and aquarium, and the Primo package, which comes with extras like the Skyfari, train, and tram. Naturally, we splurged for the Primo package because, well, who wants to walk when it's 90 degrees outside?

The Skyfari was a relaxing cable car ride that gave us a bird's-eye view of rhinos, zebras, and giraffes. We spent the rest of the day wandering through the zoo, admiring the beautifully landscaped exhibits. While the Omaha Zoo was impressive, having been to other top zoos like San Diego and Fort Worth, I wasn't entirely convinced it deserved the #1 title. But, hey, Nebraska doesn't have a lot to brag about, so I'll let them have this win.

Earlier that year, I visited the Brevard Zoo in Florida, which had some standout experiences—like ziplining and walking among kangaroos in an open exhibit with no barriers. After that, even Omaha's stellar zoo couldn't top Brevard in my book.

No trip to Omaha would be complete without trying a Reuben sandwich. There's an ongoing debate over whether the Reuben was invented in Omaha or New York. Having already sampled the NY version, it was time to try the Nebraska contender. We went to Crescent Moon, the top-rated spot for Reubens. While it was a decent sandwich, I was left underwhelmed. Sorry, Omaha, but the Big Apple wins this round. Despite the sandwich letdown, Omaha turned out to be a surprisingly fun and memorable weekend getaway.

Would I go again? Maybe. Is it at the top of my travel list? Probably not. But if I'm ever in the mood for friendly folks, a lively downtown, and a football game, I know where to go.

Tips for Visiting Nebraska:

- Want to catch a Huskers game? Check out resale tickets early, and don't forget to bring a clear bag—it's a dry stadium, so if you plan on drinking, do it before or after the game.
- September is warm, but the fall season would likely offer cooler temps and a more enjoyable experience before winter hits.
- Explore downtown Omaha. It's full of charming spots to eat, shop, and wander.
- Lincoln and Omaha cover 80% of the population, so by visiting both, you're essentially seeing all of Nebraska!

EXPERIENCE #36: HONORED THE PAST AT THE OKC MEMORIAL

The year I turned 50 was the same year my son, AJ, turned 30. AJ was adopted from Russia when he was 10, and somehow, he kept getting older until—poof—he was 30 years old. For his milestone birthday weekend, my daughter, granddaughter, and I made the trip to Kansas to celebrate with him. My daughter decided to head out earlier than I did and return later, so we took separate cars. To get from Dallas, Texas, to Kansas, you drive through Oklahoma. Growing up in Arizona with its stunning mountains, the drive through Oklahoma and Kansas (which I've now done twice) isn't exactly a scenic delight. Sorry to my friends in Oklahoma and Kansas, but it's true. I still love you.

On Saturday, July 13th, we took AJ to Top Golf to celebrate. While we were there, the news broke that Donald Trump had been shot at during a rally speech. Now, no matter what side of the political aisle you're on, shooting at someone is never okay (right Ralphie?). We were all in shock but relieved that the attempt wasn't successful (the shooter was a 20-year-old). I digress.

After a weekend of celebrating AJ and enjoying breakfast with his beautiful wife Megan and her family, it was time for me to head home. Since I was passing through Oklahoma City again on the way back, I decided to stop by the OKC Memorial and Museum.

For those unfamiliar with the Memorial, it was built to honor the victims of the Oklahoma City bombing on April 19, 1995. Timothy McVeigh, another person angry with the government (noticing a pattern here?), decided to make a big statement by blowing up the Alfred P. Murrah Federal Building. The attack killed 168 people, including children.

As you walk onto the grounds of the memorial, you're greeted by two large gates on each side. One side reads 9:01, and the other reads 9:03. The bombing occurred at 9:02. The 9:01 gate symbolizes innocence, while the 9:03 gate represents hope and healing.

Also, outside the museum, near the gates, is a grassy area with 168 chairs arranged in nine rows, representing both the people who lost their lives and the floors of the federal building that was destroyed. Seeing it all displayed was incredibly moving.

Inside the museum, there are two floors. One floor covers what was happening in the world, the country, and specifically in OKC on that fateful day, along with some background on Timothy McVeigh. The other floor focuses on the aftermath—what happened after the bombing, the legal proceedings, and a memorial to the victims.

One thing that really stuck with me was a quote from the judge (I'm paraphrasing here). He pointed out that the very government Timothy McVeigh was so angry with was the same government that ensured he had a fair trial. Oh, the irony.

I left the memorial deep in thought (and in tears) about how many people have paid the price for someone else's anger. It served as a powerful reminder for us all to put a little more love and peace into the world.

Would I do this experience again? The memorial is so beautifully done, and I'm grateful I took the time to visit. However, once is probably enough for me.

Tips if you want to try it:

- It's worth the $20 (at the time of this writing) to go inside the museum and get a deeper understanding of the events of that day. Your admission also supports the museum.
- Do some extra homework: Many documentaries have been made about this event, so if you want some additional background information, they're worth checking out.

EXPERIENCE #37: RELISHED A PRIVATE CHEF PREPARED MEAL WITH FRIENDS

I love delicious food—like, a lot. I also love my friends. So, when you mix the two together, pure joy ensues.

I am incredibly lucky to have so many wonderful people in my life, and one group that holds a particularly special place in my heart is my lifetime friends, affectionately referred to as "lifers." We are a group of seven women who have been friends for decades—two of whom I've known since first grade! The rest of the crew formed in our high school years. We've lived states apart, experienced all kinds of life changes, but no matter how much time passes, we always pick right back up where we left off.

Over a decade ago, we started a tradition: every other year, we take a trip together. With raising kids, navigating careers, and dealing with life's endless to-do list, finding a common weekend was always a challenge. But we made it happen! San Diego, Flagstaff, Colorado, and

Huntington Beach have been some of our past destinations. This year's trip was extra special—it was our 50th birthday celebration trip! We chose Lake Tahoe, a beautiful place I had never been before.

After some deliberation, we settled on a stunning Airbnb with a view of the lake. Katie, one of the planners in our group, had a surprise up her sleeve. The rental offered concierge services (boujee, right?!), and Katie, along with a couple of the other girls, secretly arranged for private chefs to prepare dinner for our first night together.

When we arrived at the house, we were a little tired from travel, but that didn't stop us from diving into hours of catching up. The chefs showed up not long after, bringing all the supplies and ingredients with them, so we didn't have to lift a finger. It was heaven. We stayed on the couch, chatting away, while they prepped everything in the kitchen. Then, the appetizers arrived! The first was heirloom bruschetta with sweet basil and Danish feta cheese, and the other was shrimp with a special garlic aioli sauce that was to die for. I'm the only non-drinker in the group, but it was still fun to watch my friends sip their wine and cocktails as we enjoyed the first bites of our special meal.

Dinner was served in the dining room, and we were delighted to see that the chefs had even taken the time to fold the napkins into roses. It was such a thoughtful touch. The meal began with warm, freshly baked bread, followed by a panzanella salad, and then came the main courses: pan-roasted sea bass, wild mushroom risotto, braced short ribs, and a side of roasted veggies. Everything was absolutely delicious. To top it all off, we were treated to a molten chocolate cake for dessert—rich, decadent, and the perfect sweet finish.

And the best part? We didn't have to wash a single dish. That, my friends, is luxury!

There's something magical about enjoying a gourmet meal in the comfort of your home (or in this case, a rental home) without having to worry about cooking or cleaning. It allowed us to focus on what truly mattered, catching up, laughing, and simply being in the moment with each other. This experience made our first night in Tahoe unforgettable. It was the perfect gift, and I'll forever be grateful for it.

Would I do this again? Absolutely! I'm not sure what my friends paid for the experience, but I'd love to return the favor one day. This is something I'd definitely consider for future trips, too.

Tips if You Want to Try This:

- Look up "experiences" on Airbnb or simply Google private chefs in your area.
- Make sure to ask if there are any dietary restrictions or preferences in your group.
- Confirm with the chef if they'll be bringing everything, including things like oven mitts, towels, and serving ware. Sometimes rentals don't have these supplies.

- If you ever get the chance to hire a private chef for a special occasion—whether it's for a trip or a staycation at home—do it! It's an experience you won't soon forget.

EXPERIENCE #38: HIKED, BIKED AND KAYAKED IN LAKE TAHOE

For years, Lake Tahoe has been sitting pretty at the top of my "must-visit" list. Since I've already ticked off all 50 states, people just assume I've been to Tahoe. I mean, why wouldn't I have? It straddles Nevada and California like a scenic overachiever, isn't far from Arizona (where I grew up), and is practically begging hikers like me to explore its endless, jaw-droppingly gorgeous trails. Maybe it's the allure of its crystal-clear waters, or perhaps it's just the Tahoe hype—it's a place that sounds so iconic, you almost feel like you've been there, even if you haven't. But alas, I hadn't yet made it. When my lifelong high school friends and I decided to make Tahoe the destination for our big 50th birthday bash, I couldn't have been more thrilled! Side note: all of them had already been to Tahoe at various points in their lives.

After a stunning (and borderline life-altering) private chef experience on our first night, we were ready to trade to tackle the great outdoors. Naturally, as the self-appointed hiking enthusiast of the group, I was put in charge of picking the trail for Day #2. Enter: Chimney Beach Trail. A quick scroll through my trusty AllTrails app, and I knew this would be the one. We piled into our rental car and set off toward the trailhead, channeling our inner Lewis and Clark, minus the whole "uncharted wilderness" ordeal. Let's be real—we were following a GPS most of the time.

The rain from the previous day had left the air smelling like a pine-scented candle, only better because it was the real deal. We couldn't resist stopping every five minutes to take pictures, which, looking back, was probably overkill. We ended up snapping about 1.2 million photos (give or take a few). Rookie mistake—we should've brought a selfie stick or a tripod to save ourselves the trouble. The trail was as beautiful as advertised—though we did manage to wander off course at one point, thanks to getting a little too wrapped up in our chatting session.

And then, BAM! Out of nowhere, I felt a sharp sting in my calf. I yelped. A yellow jacket had stung me—*through my leggings!* Seriously, of all the places to get stung, right? I immediately plopped down on the ground, while my friend Sue went into full MacGyver mode, dumping water on the sting with the precision of a field medic. Meanwhile, Vanessa, ever the quick thinker, started slathering mud on the sting like a Girl Scout. Honestly, I was impressed by their survival skills. Just then, a couple wandered by, and I figured it couldn't hurt to ask if they had any first-aid supplies. To my surprise—and eternal gratitude—they did! Armed with a cleaning pad, Neosporin, and a Band-Aid, I was good as new (well, mostly). Bless those random hikers. Curse that yellow-jacket!

My leg was still a in fully "stinging" mode, but I powered through. We managed to finish the hike, though we had to cut it short to make our 4 p.m. dinner reservation at the famous Wolf Restaurant (the ownder is the lead in the ever-dramatic reality series Vanderpump Rules). Yes, you read that right—4 *p.m.* I know, we're officially in early-bird territory. Move over, senior citizens, there's a new crew in town. The only options for dining were 4pm or 10pm. We knew our limits. 4 p.m for the win. Dinner at The Wolf on the opposite side of the lake was delicious, and honestly, after that hike (and the sting drama), we were more than ready to indulge in some fine dining.

The next day, the group was divided. Half of us wanted to go on a bike ride, while the other half decided to kick back and relax on the deck of our Airbnb, soaking in the views of Lake Tahoe. There's no wrong answer when it comes to things to do in Tahoe, so we were all winning. The four of us who opted for the bike ride rented electric bikes from a great little place called Tahoe MultiSport. They also do glass-bottom kayak tours, which I mentally bookmarked for my next trip because *yes, please*.

We started our ride in a gorgeous neighborhood called Incline Village, along a road appropriately named Lakeshore Drive. As we pedaled along, we were surrounded by massive pine trees and multi-million-dollar homes that looked like they belonged in a travel magazine. Eventually, Lakeshore led us to a bike path that wound its way up the mountain, offering us breathtaking views of Emerald Cove and Sand Harbor. It was like riding through a postcard—vivid blue lake, towering trees, and majestic mountains everywhere you looked. Naturally, we had to stop *again* to take even more pictures, because when you're faced with vistas like that, you just can't help yourself.

After a quick bite to eat in Sand Harbor, we hopped back on the bikes and discovered an area called the Flume Trail. Now, this was no leisurely paved path—this was a real mountain trail, rugged and wild. And let me tell you, this is where we *really* leaned into the "electric" part of our electric bikes. Without that extra boost, I'm not sure we would've made it through. By the time we returned the bikes, we were both exhausted and exhilarated, completely in awe of the natural beauty surrounding us.

The last active day of our trip had fewer participants —some of the girls had transitioned into full-on "drink on the patio with a view" mode, which, let's be honest, is a totally valid way to experience Tahoe. But three of us were still itching for some adventure and actually wanted to get out on the water. Now, let me preface this by saying: I am not made for paddleboarding. Balancing on a glorified surfboard while trying not to face-plant into the lake isn't exactly my forte. However, my two friends were practically born with paddles in their hands, so they hopped on their boards with all the grace of seasoned pros. I, on the other hand, opted for the much more "sit down and don't tip over" approach —kayaking.

By "around the lake," I mean a tiny, picturesque sliver of it. Lake Tahoe is *massive*—we're talking 1,645 feet deep and covering 191 square miles. It's not the kind of place you casually circle in a kayak while humming the theme from *Moana*. And because it's so deep, we took exactly zero valuables with us. Drop something in Tahoe, and you might as well kiss it goodbye, because it's not coming back. Not even Jacques Cousteau could retrieve your sunglasses from those depths.

We were incredibly lucky with the weather during our trip. It only rained on our arrival day, and after that, it was sunshine and blue skies all the way. The lake itself, while crystal-clear and gorgeous, is *cold*. But surprisingly, I didn't have a full-blown *Titanic* moment every time the water splashed on me. You know the scene—Jack sinking into the icy abyss while Rose dramatically clings to a door (which, side note, was *totally* big enough for two). Luckily, it wasn't quite that dramatic for me, although I did get a few refreshing splashes that reminded me this wasn't the Mediterranean.

We piddled and paddled out on the lake for about an hour before we decided to visit our friends on the patio, arriving with the trifecta badge of exploring Tahoe by foot, bike, and water.

So, would I visit Tahoe again? In a heartbeat. It's stunning, peaceful, and has adventure around every corner.

If you're planning an active vacation to Lake Tahoe, here are a few tips to make the most of it:

1. **Bring a tripod or selfie stick.** Trust me, your arms will thank you.
2. **Pack for all kinds of weather.** The weather can change quickly, so layers are your best friend.
3. **Keep a first-aid kit handy.** You never know when nature will throw a yellow jacket your way.
4. **Hydrate and Snack Smart**: Bring plenty of water and some healthy snacks. Staying fueled will keep your energy up during those long hikes or bike rides.
5. **Check Local Trail Conditions**: Before heading out, check for any trail closures or conditions. Websites and local visitor centers can provide up-to-date info to help you plan your route.
6. **Try Sunrise or Sunset Adventures**: The views during these times are breathtaking, and you'll avoid the crowds while enjoying cooler temperatures.
7. **Explore Hidden Beaches**: Don't just stick to the popular spots; take the time to find some lesser-known beaches for a quieter paddleboarding or kayaking experience. You might discover a hidden gem!
8. **Don't miss the Flume Trail.** It's challenging but so worth it—just make sure you've got an electric bike to help with those uphill climbs!

EXPERIENCE #38: DID A HEAD STAND IN YOGA

I've been a certified 200-hour yoga teacher since 2014. When I first enrolled in the certification program (which took nine months), I was only a sort of yoga lover. My favorite teacher, Diane, was the only one I attended regularly. She taught a class on Sundays called "Slow Sundays," the best feel-good, slow yoga you could imagine. I wasn't into the sweaty hot yoga or the advanced stuff. At the time, I was teaching five Zumba classes a week and was only looking to chill.

In 2014, after two years of Slow Sundays and some major challenges with my kids, I decided to enroll in a yoga certification program. I had no idea why, other than that my life was stressful, and it sounded like I could have some more Slow Sundays in my future.

The first class I attended, the instructor asked us to teach a 30-minute yoga class. I tried to remember what Diane had taught, but nothing was flowing (literally and figuratively). I think the patient yoga instructor was wondering why I even bothered to sign up for the class with such limited knowledge. But I persevered, and after nine months (equaling 200 hours), I was certified to teach basic yoga.

My first few classes were at a Chinese Sunday School. It was a class for the parents while their kids were learning Chinese. I was decent, and they were kind. It was a helpful place to start.

Over the next few years, I taught yoga here and there, but never consistently. Whenever I looked for a class to take, I was always on the hunt for that Slow Sunday vibe. I taught yoga several times for a company that offers yoga vacations at resorts and subbed a few yoga classes at the gyms where I teach Zumba. It was usually in emergency situations, and some of the students were happy just to have a teacher, while others would bust out a few crazy yoga poses and then leave. Did I mention I'm very basic?

Another aspect of yoga I've never fully connected with is flexibility. I know how important it is to stay limber as we age, but I've found my body tightening up more each year. I always marveled at the people in my classes who could wrap their legs around their heads or do poses that looked like a circus demo.

Fast forward to July 2024. It was a tough month. Usually, when things get tough, I know the tools to calm my nervous system: walks, journaling, breathing, service, gratitude. But nothing was pulling me out of the stress. I had an eye twitch that wouldn't go away. I found a retreat in early August a couple of hours from home that I signed up for to help (more of that in the next chapter), but the weekend before, I had nothing planned. So, I searched Facebook for events and found another yoga retreat just 10 minutes away, at the same place where I'd hosted a retreat before. Kismet! It was also sponsored by the non-profit Yoga Health Institute, so the price was lower than the average retreat. I signed up, and two days later, I was there.

Ricky, the organizer and master yoga teacher, was phenomenal. He shared how he started yoga 20 years ago to get off speed. This led him to seek out the best teachers around, and eventually, he got certified and opened several studios around Dallas-Fort Worth. For one of our practice sessions, Ricky introduced headstands. I laughed. I rolled my eyes. No way, mister. Not a chance I'm trying that. I admired the people around me who went for it, and I sat it out. The following day, we had a slower yoga practice—still a lot of movement, but not as intense as the day before. At the very end, Ricky brought back the headstands. Oh brother. Not a chance.

Then, I watched Ricky help one of the other girls slowly get into the pose, and suddenly, I wanted to do this. What had come over me? I don't know! But as Ricky walked by, I heard myself say, "I want to try." He came over and talked me through it, and I must have said to him no less than 14 times, "Don't let go." Slowly, ever so slowly, I was there! I was doing a freaking headstand! It was an unexpected victory in a practice that teaches you to release the ego.

Would I do this experience again? I think so, but only with assistance from a yoga teacher.

Tips if you want to try it:

- Make sure you don't have any cervical issues. For real. Stay away from this if you have neck problems.
- Do it with a yoga teacher holding and guiding you. That support makes all the difference.
- There are preparatory poses to learn and practice before attempting a headstand. I recommend mastering those and working your way up to the pose.

EXPERIENCE #39: FOUND MY ANIMAL ZEN AT A WILDLIFE YOGA RETREAT

I got dumped. Technically, it was a mutual dump. But this one stung more than most—this was the special guy I was supposed to go to Paris with to watch the Olympics. He loved to travel as much as me. Talk about an extra ouch. I was in desperate need of some serious self-care.

A friend of mine had once mentioned a place called Oak Meadow Ranch in Texas. She and her husband had stayed there for their anniversary, and she couldn't stop raving about it. The ranch was home to some unique animals, and she fell in love with the place. I tucked the idea away for the future, following their Facebook page in the meantime.

So, imagine my surprise when, just days after the breakup, an advertisement popped up on my feed for the first-ever wildlife yoga retreat at Oak Meadow Ranch. It wasn't cheap, and I wasn't sure if I could get the time off work, but before I could even think about those practicalities, I found myself booking a spot. Of course I was going to go!

Oak Meadow Ranch is in Valley View, Texas, a place I had never heard of, even though I've lived in the Dallas-Fort Worth area since 2003. It's less than 90 minutes from my house but feels worlds away—remote, serene, and surrounded by horse farms. As I drove up to the ranch, I was greeted by an enthusiastic staff member (I later learned that all of their staff members are this level of fantastic). After signing a waiver and parking, they loaded my suitcase onto a golf cart and whisked me away to my room.

I had chosen this room for one very specific reason: Puzzles. And no, I'm not talking about the kind we all did during the great lockdown of 2020. Puzzles is a 17-year-old giraffe. The building I stayed in has two stories and four separate rooms. I was downstairs in the Wagoneer, a room that was adorably western and well-appointed. Inside, there was a bag of goodies, including a journal and necklace from our retreat host, plus water in the fridge. But the real magic was what lay just beyond the curtains.

I pulled them back to reveal a large window with Puzzles standing right there. It was the kind of moment that makes you smile, cry, and giggle all at once. Beside the large window was a small one with a cover that opened—a little hatch where you could feed Puzzles from your bedroom. They provided carrots and lettuce, and soon, Puzzles was at my window, his enormous tongue reaching out for the treats. I was in heaven. Screw Paris.

My room was also next to the kangaroos. Though I couldn't feed them, it was still pretty cool to watch them hop around, especially since there was a baby roo among them. Bunnies hung out with the kangaroos, adopting a "birds of a feather" mentality, I suppose.

The retreat officially kicked off at 4 p.m. with a charcuterie board sprinkled with edible glitter (I quickly learned that sparkly things are a theme here, adding a level of next-level bouje to the experience). Slowly, the other participants gathered—seven of us in total, including our yoga teacher—and we made casual conversation.

After that, we walked over to the red barn for our first night of yoga and breathwork. I was especially excited about this evening. It wasn't just the cute setup of fake candles, mats, blocks, and bolsters that had me eager. Nor was it the fact that we had a camel on one side of the barn and two water buffalo on the other side, casually watching us move. It wasn't even the breathing and body movements, although those were wonderful too. No, the thing I was most looking forward to was meeting and holding Sir Winston. Not a future boyfriend, but a sloth.

I had always dreamed of getting up close and personal with a sloth, but I never imagined it would actually happen. Sloths typically aren't human-oriented, but Sir Winston was an exception. He was gentle and peaceful, and when the caretaker brought him into our yoga session, she placed him with Heather, one of the other retreat participants. Sir Winston sat there in a totally zen state. I was next. This is why I had come here.

Sitting on a bolster, the animal keeper instructed me to support Sir Winston underneath. His arms wrapped around me in a hug, and I melted. Tears streamed down my cheeks. In somatics (body/emotion work), there's this thing called co-regulation. When you hug someone for at least 30 seconds, it can regulate your emotions. Sir Winston did that for me. When it was time to pass him to the next person, I felt a deep sense of peace and joy. Anything that came after Puzzles and Sir Winston was just icing on an already beautiful cake.

After yoga, we headed to the wild side of the ranch where there are cats, lemurs, and more. We sat around a firepit, chatting for a while, and I realized that these special women were gifts to me. This was exactly where I was supposed to be.

The next day began with a delightful breakfast followed by more yoga. We had a bit of free time, during which I did some work (I had been at my job for only two months and was lucky to have been granted the time off). Then, it was time for horse therapy.

Horses are beautiful, and I love looking at them, but there's a reason I failed every test at Girl Scout Horse Camp at age 9. Horses and I just aren't meant for each other, especially not at 2 p.m. in the 103-degree Texas summer sun. Horse therapy involved brushing the horses and walking them while trying to prevent them from eating grass. I was kind of done with that activity early on.

After horse therapy, I opted for an extra activity— swimming with otters. I mean, come on, how often do you get a chance to do that? The otters' names were Harry P. Otter and Ron Weasley (I think that was the second name, though I'm not totally sure). These little characters were funny, smart, and full of energy! Me and two other ladies who chose this activity sat in a very small pool while the otters joined us. They were crazy, swimming into the pockets of my shorts, into another woman's bathing suit, and into the top of the third. These otters had no boundaries. For almost an hour, we played with them—it was partially glorious, partially exhausting, and totally worth it.

After otter time, we quickly changed for yoga, and towards the end of the session, they brought in a tiny monkey-like creature that crawled and jumped around us. Very cute! Then, we moved on to dinner.

After dinner, we had some free time, and I'm going to admit something very vulnerable here—no matter how amazing the experience was, my mind didn't completely shut off. There were moments when I thought about the Olympics and the guy. In a moment of weakness, I sent him a text about where I was and what I was doing. His response? "Cool. I'm on my way to Europe (first class, of course) to see the Olympics." And he wasn't alone. It was a gut punch. I'm human, after all, and it was a sucky moment. My mind was struggling.

At the end of the day, we went back to the barn for a gorgeous sound bath. If you've never done a sound bath, it typically involves sound bowls, a gong, and a few other instruments. This sound bath lady had it all—like 10 different sound devices. And she was good! But my mind wouldn't shut off. After the sound bath, I went to bed and realized I had to make a conscious choice moving forward about where I let my thoughts go. So I did. The next day, I felt a shift—kind of like when you dread bad news, but the anticipation is worse than the actual news. Once it comes, you can finally accept it and move forward. That's how I started the next day. Well, that and also feeding Puzzles.

The final day, we had breakfast and then our yoga session was actually inside the lemur enclosure, as opposed to the lemurs being brought to us. It was hard to stay focused on yoga with them bouncing around, but it was pretty neat to see them up close again.

I said my our goodbyes to the wonderful group of women after that, and I left this magical place to head home. I wasn't feeling great health-wise when I left—I thought the animals and dust from the ground had made me sick, but it turned out to be COVID. Still, totally worth every minute of being there.

Would I do this experience again? Absolutely! When I say this place is magical, I mean it. The animals are so well cared for, the rooms are beautiful, the food is good, and the staff is incredible. Combining all of that with a yoga retreat is next-level amazing. So yes, in one form or another, I will be back.

Tips If You Want to Try It

- Decide if you want to go for the day or stay the night: Both options have their charm, but staying overnight offers a deeper experience.

- Check room availability: If you can, book one of the giraffe rooms. If not, the Silos is another great option—beautifully decorated and unique.
- Plan your activities: If you're going for the day, choose the activities you want to do in advance. The website lists all available options, including camel rides and otter swims.
- Consider the yoga retreat: If you're into yoga, the retreat is a totally different and wonderful experience, but it's not for everyone.

Experience #43: Participate in a Drum Circle

Experience #44: Go to Omaha, Nebraska to Visit the Top Zoo in the Nation

Experience #45: Lake Tahoe

Experience #46: Colorado Springs-Nudist Resort

Experience #47-Cheesemaking Class

Experience #48-Hot Air Balloon Ride

Experience #49 Go to a live TedX Talk

Experience #50: Write and Publish a Book

UNTITLED

Experience #40: Stood in Awe at the Beauty of Acadia National Park

EXPERIENCE #41: MET WITH A FINANCIAL PLANNER AND DINED MY WAY THROUGH FINANCIAL WISDOM

If there was anything I have spent extra time avoiding, it was thinking about my financial situation for retirement. I figured if I just didn't think about it, then when I turned 67, magically, funds would show up in my bank account and I would be able to enjoy a life of luxury for the next 30 years. Carpe Diem!

Then, post my divorce, when funds were very tight, I learned how not so great it feels to be constantly busting my butt to make ends meet. It took a few years to be in a place where I could start a 401k at work, and I when I did, I closed my eyes and imagined that retirement money would naturally flow in. Except it doesn't work like that. Sadly.

I walk that tight line between saving and enjoying. I want to save. I have an emergency savings account thankfully. I also want to enjoy life as we are not promised tomorrow. So, I live life as fully as possible, realizing that both sides have value. I think though, if we are talking ratio, I have given 75% to living fully and 25% to saving. Retirement at this time looks a little murky.

When I was at the Wildlife Yoga Retreat, I did something totally spontaneous. One of the participants, Georgia, a wonderfully kind and warm lady in her early 70's, told me that Allen, the owner of Oak Meadow Ranch, is her Financial Planner. She said he did wonderful things with her money, so much so that I learned she funded the building where the giraffe currently lives. All hail Puzzles and Georgia!

One retreat day at lunch, Allen joined us, and I asked him about financial planning. He offered to talk to me about it, and we set up a time post my facial at the retreat to come by (I told you; I really do try to live life fully). So, before dinner, we met, and he shared with me about how he does his planning and what I could do. My favorite part about what he said was that he schedules a quarterly phone call with each client to update them on the progress of their accounts. That translates to me this: I don't have to pay attention until I get that phone call. Winning!

Since I have four 401k accounts from different companies I have worked at, we had to have a phone call to request a check from each of them and then when the checks were delivered to my house, one of the people that work for Allen came to pick them up. My adventures in financial freedom at fifty (ok, 67) were becoming a reality with taking this first step. Allen now had my money, and I was hopeful he could turn me into a millionaire or at least a thousandaire.

After all this happened, my friend Kane reached out to me to see if I wanted to go with him to a financial planning seminar at a steakhouse, a really nice one in our city. It was a chance to eat really good food so that you would then trust them with your money. I told Kane that I had just recently gotten a financial planner, but he told me they didn't know that and to come along. Free salmon! I am saving money already.

I had gotten mailers about these free seminars for various services in the past, but I had never gone to any of them. I didn't know what to expect really. My friend Kane met me at the restaurant, and we went into the bar to split an appetizer while we waited for the seminar. The seminar was held at a restaurant called Steve Fields. It was fancy, darkly lit, and very nice. The room in the back of the restaurant lacked the appeal like the rest of the place, but perhaps a big TV and a ready to go PowerPoint can do that. There were two financial advisors there. One sat at a table while the other one (Bob) presented.

While he was about to get started, they brought in the salads. Meh. I know this isn't a book with restaurant reviews, but as a public service announcement, good salads are ruined by bad dressing. I digress. Bob began the presentation by bringing up a graphic that showed all the areas of finances we have to be aware of when we retire: Cashflow, Investment Management, Social Security, Insurance, Medicare, Tax Planning, Estate Planning, Large Purchases, and Recreation. Reading that list caused my anxiety to creep up quite a bit. So many areas, so little funds.

I stopped listening to him, and let my eyes look around the room. Who else attended these things? Most of the people in there were in their 50s and beyond. Some were already retired. There were a lot of couples. I imagine the mailer was sent to married couples to attend together. Kane's wife couldn't make it, so I got to eat the salmon on her behalf. It also seemed as though the people there fell in the financially middle class and above category. The firm did their homework.

I focused back into the presentation. They continued to share all the areas that we need to save in and what would happen if we didn't (like what happened to the original owner of the Miami Dolphins). He wrapped up the hour-long presentation and said they would be coming around to answer questions as well as setup phone call times for anyone interested in learning more. Nobody at our table said yes, but I am not sure the success they had in the rest of the room. Our dinner was delivered, and we ate and chatted as the presenter and other financial planner circled the room in hopes to make connections. They sent in two people who came around to set up calls. When we all said no, their response was dessert will be served. Not even the carrot cake could hook me in.

Would I try this again? I am glad that I found a solid and experienced financial planner (Allen) and feel like my 401ks are now safely in the same place with supervision. As far as attending the Financial Seminar Dinner, it would depend on if I was hungry or not. Is the meal worth the time and sales presentation (just ask anyone who has sat through time shares). I supposed if the presenter was really good and informative, it would be worth a go.

Tips If You Want to Try It

- Look at Eventbrite to see if there are any type of events like this.
- Ask your trusted friends who they use for their financial planners and if they are satisfied with their service or not. Interview the ones that got a thumbs up and see if you find a match
- Go to the library (or Amazon) and get some books on financial planning that encompass all the topics that Bob shared above. If anything, it is eye opening to consider your finances and know some steps to take (even baby steps count!)

EXPERIENCE #42: DUCKED AND WEAVED IN A FENCING CLASS

Medieval Times wasn't exactly a shining example of humanity at its best—think Black Plague and the Crusades. However, out of that chaotic era emerged the refined art of fencing. My only exposure to the sport before this was watching The Princess Bride, where Inigo Montoya shows off his fencing prowess, seeking revenge on the man with six fingers. So, when I spotted an introduction to fencing class on Facebook Events, I was hooked! It was 10:17 AM on a Sunday morning, and the class was starting at 11:00 AM. Despite still being snug in bed, I jumped up and donned my best fencing attire. To be honest, I had no clue what actual fencing gear looked like, so I went with yoga pants and a black top—trying to channel my inner fencer.

The class was held at a park in Richardson, Texas. By the time I arrived, they were already well into a class that preceded the introductory one. The school, Valiant: School of Arms, had a serious vibe. I approached the small group of about nine people, all of whom were dressed far more appropriately than my yoga-clad self (and, to be fair, I was the only woman there). I inquired if this was indeed the introduction class and was directed to Eric, the owner.

Eric looked every bit the part of a Medieval Times fencer—long hair, a ruggedly handsome face, and attire reminiscent of the 1400s. He greeted me warmly, shook my hand, and welcomed me to the class. After signing in (no waiver required), we dove right in. Eric handed me a pair of gloves and a sword, the sharp end covered with thick tape for safety. I appreciated that we were keeping things non-lethal. He demonstrated how to hold the sword, then gathered the group for a salute—head, heart, and honor, I believe.

Since I was the only newbie, Eric partnered with me. He would demonstrate a skill, and then we'd practice it in pairs. We used a rapier sword, and Eric called over Timmy, instructing him to "put the tip in." I had to stifle a "That's what she said" joke—clearly, I'm not mature enough for fencing.

We practiced a few moves whose names escape me now, and then we strapped on helmets. I felt like a total badass—albeit a sweaty one, given that it was September 1st and summer was still blazing. My fencing moves apparently included some Zumba flair, which looked hilarious and would likely have been deadly in a real medieval duel.

At the end of class, we did the salute one last time, and I asked if we could take a group photo. The group was incredibly sweet and agreed—who was this strange woman in black, after all? I chatted with them afterward and asked what kind of people are usually drawn to fencing. Their response? Fans of Dungeons and Dragons.

Would I try this again? Probably not. While I enjoyed the experience and found everyone welcoming, it wasn't quite my thing. Plus, my wrist and arm were definitely feeling it afterward!

Tips If You Want to Try It

- Find a Local School: Look up fencing schools near you and start with a beginner's class.
- Try Before You Buy: Test out a class to see if fencing is right for you before investing in your own equipment.
- Embrace the Challenge: If you're looking to push yourself with something new, give fencing a shot. Just remember, Inigo Montoya would be proud of your adventurous spirit!

EXPERIENCE #43: FELT THE
BEAT IN A DRUM CIRCLE

For about a year, I had been seeing advertisements for drum circles, and I wasn't quite sure what to expect. My first thought was, "Is this a group of drummers gathering to showcase their skills, or does it literally mean a bunch of people sitting in a circle, drumming away together?" It turns out, it's the latter—just a bunch of people with drums sitting in a circle, playing. But the simplicity of it intrigued me, and I decided it was worth experiencing at least once.

A friend of mine from Tampa had mentioned that her mom goes to drum circles on the beach, not to play but just to observe. Apparently, the events could gather hundreds of people all drumming together. The idea of so many people coming together for music-making struck me as fascinating. I love the idea of community and connection through music, and even though I'm not much of a drummer myself, I thought, "Why not?" Plus, my friend "B" was going through a rough patch in life and seemed to need a pick-me-up. I invited him to come along, hoping that this event would offer him a new experience and maybe lift his spirits. At the very least, I could provide a friendly ear. As for having a good time? Well, that was up in the air, but I was hopeful.

We decided to attend a drum circle in Richardson, Texas, at a local brewery called Four Bullets Brewery. They hold this event once a month, and the setting was unique—tucked in the old part of town with the DART rail rumbling overhead. It gave the space a bit of character, almost like you were in some artsy, off-the-beaten-path neighborhood that locals keep secret. We arrived right when the event started at 7 p.m., though people were still slowly filtering in. "B" grabbed a beer, and I opted for water (staying hydrated while drumming seemed like a good plan). We didn't know what to expect, so we waited around, taking in the scene.

The lead drummer, a man named Michael Kenny, had been involved in the drumming community for over 30 years. I could tell he was a beloved figure from the way people greeted him as they arrived. He had this calm, welcoming presence about him, which was reassuring for newbies like us. He provided plenty of spare drums for those who didn't bring their own (like us), as well as a variety of percussion instruments like maracas, tambourines, and a few other things I didn't even recognize. Michael explained that he was a music therapist and that these drum circles were more than just about making noise—they were about releasing pent-up energy and emotions. Apparently, drumming together could be a form of therapy, a way to de-stress and let go.

We all formed a circle (no surprise there), and each person sat in front of their chosen drum. Most of the drums were djembe-style, the African hand drums that produce deep, resonant sounds. These weren't the kind of drums you'd see at a rock concert—no electric sets or drum kits. Some drums were massive, taller than a person, standing on the floor. Others, like the one "B" and I had, were smaller, about two feet tall, and tucked between our legs. It felt authentic, like something you'd see in a cultural celebration or a tribal gathering. Michael instructed us to just start playing, not worrying about rhythm or whether we were in sync with anyone else. The idea was to feel free, let loose, and not get bogged down by technicalities. So, we did.

It started as a cacophony of random beats—everyone doing their own thing. Some people had mallets to drum with, while others, like Benjy and me, used the palms of their hands. After a while, though, something magical began to happen. The randomness started to merge into this beautiful, rhythmic flow. People weren't copying each other, but somehow it all blended together. The drumming took on a life of its own, and we became part of a collective sound. It was oddly meditative, even though I wasn't entirely sure I was doing it "right" (if there even was a right way).

The crowd was a mix of all kinds of people—hippies, music lovers, and those just there for a good time. Everyone was welcoming and warm. There was a definite free-spirited vibe in the air, enhanced by the unmistakable scent of weed that wafted through the group from time to time. A few people got up to dance, swaying to the beats. One man had brought his own wooden flutes and played them intermittently, blending their ethereal sound with the drumming, and occasionally taking a break to puff on something. The mix of sounds, movements, and the easygoing atmosphere felt like a throwback to a different era. It was a little Woodstock, a little Burning Man—right there in the middle of Richardson, Texas.

I looked over at "B", who had really found his groove. He was totally absorbed in the drumming, smiling and nodding his head to his own beat. It was the first time I'd seen him look that relaxed, and it made me glad I'd dragged him along. There's something about the rhythm that seems to reach people on a deeper level, beyond just the physical act of hitting a drum. Maybe it was therapeutic after all.

After two hours of continuous drumming, I was starting to feel it in my arms, and I could tell I was about done. The event was free, but there was a tip jar, so we made sure to throw in some money before we left. We waved goodbye to Michael and the others, with the sounds of the final song fading as we walked away.

"B" left in a noticeably better mood, which made the whole evening worthwhile. Sometimes, it's the simplest things—like banging on a drum for a couple of hours—that can shift a person's energy. Drumming really can be a form of therapy, it seems.

Would I do it again? Probably not. I'm glad I tried it,

but it's not something I'd go out of my way to repeat. That said, if a friend really wanted to go, I wouldn't say no. It was a unique experience, just not one that's calling me back.

Tips if you want to try it:

- I found this drum circle event on Facebook and Eventbrite, so those are good places to start.
- You can also do a quick Google search for "Drum Circles near me" and see what comes up.
- Check ahead of time to see if it's okay to just observe or if participation is required.
- Bring water, be open to the experience, and don't worry if you're not musically inclined. The point is to enjoy the moment. You might just find a surprising sense of peace in the rhythm.

UNTITLED

Experience #45: Savored a Community Meal on the Streets of Downtown Plano

EXPERIENCE #46: BARED IT ALL AT A NUDIST RESORT

Times in my life I've been naked with a bunch of strangers?

Zero.

Until now.

Let me clarify upfront: I did *not* start an OnlyFans account or join a swingers group. This was different.

I had a list of my 10 final things left on my "Year I Turned 50" list, and I read it aloud to a friend. His simple reply? "You need to do something way outside your comfort zone. You're not pushing yourself. Do better, Staci."

Okay, maybe he didn't actually say "Do better, Staci," but I translated it to that—and then dove deep.

Look, I've done some pretty wild things outside my comfort zone before. In 7th grade, we all peed in Ziploc bags at a slumber party and left them on a neighbor's porch with a "Merry Christmas" note (sorry, neighbor). I tried out for the boys' basketball team in middle school (puberty was just setting in, so fear hadn't quite caught up). Ran for student council in high school (won twice, lost once), tried out for cheerleading (three times made it, once didn't). In college, I changed religions, went on a mission to a country where I barely spoke the language, and married a man I hadn't really dated (he lived abroad). Oh, and I adopted four kids from Russia. I also strated three businesses and have traveled the world solo.

Take that "push yourself out of your comfort zone" and shove it.

And yet...he was kind of right. If I was being honest with myself, I needed to go next-level. It was time to watch bird-watching off the list (not that there is anything wrong with it). We brainstormed, and the idea of a nudist resort came up. I shrieked "NO WAY!" And then...I thought how much of a stretch this would be for me. I accepted the challenge.

I know what you're thinking. Actually, I have no idea what you're thinking, but I'll share what I was thinking and what everyone else I told this to was thinking:

- Will it be hard to not stare at people's parts?
- Is it fully naked, or just boobs out and bottoms on?
- What if it's cold?
- Is this, like, a sex party?
- Probably just old people, right?

I'll answer all those questions and more, but first, some background.

I knew I wanted to do this out of state—seeing someone from my neighborhood or my Zumba class while naked wasn't ideal. The closest place with affordable tickets and a nudist resort? Colorado.

Colorado has a handful of clothing-optional resorts and hot springs, so after a search on Google, I settled on Mountain Air Ranch (MAR)—a *family* nudist resort just outside Littleton. This ranch, nestled on 150 acres, has been around for nearly 90 years. There's hiking, a pool, jacuzzi, game rooms, tennis courts, and even bocce ball. You can stay on-site or bring an RV. It's like summer camp with less clothes!

I flew to Colorado the night before, and on the day of, I shaved all the important places and told myself cellulite is just cheese angels kissing my body. I arrived for my 10 a.m. tour, not knowing what to expect. Walking into the office, everyone was clothed. Did I mess up the address? Was I in the right place?

Then *she* walked in—Nudy Judy (name changed for anonymity). Nudy Judy (NJ) was a bubbly 66-year-old with a floral robe, loosely open but leaving nothing to the imagination. Okay, I'm in the right place.

NJ enthusiastically handed me paperwork. They have a code of conduct: no public sexual activity, no illegal drugs, no drunkenness, and watch your language (because kids might be there). It's basically church...if church were naked. Photography is banned in common areas—gotta keep some mystery alive, I guess. I signed the papers, got my gate pass, and off we went on a golf cart tour with NJ and another couple.

First "Whoa!" moment? Driving by the tennis courts where four people were playing *naked* pickleball. My first thought? "Those unsupported boobs must be bouncing all over." (Okay, fine, that was my second thought. The first was, "Oh my gosh, naked pickleball!")

Then we cruised by a guy sitting in his lawn chair, stark naked, while another group was working in a common kitchen area. Casual as can be. NJ shared some hilarious stories about her time there, including how she first came on her 30th anniversary trip *without* her husband. She went home, filed for divorce, and never looked back. That was the day she lost her "nudegenity." Sixteen years later, she's an institution at this place.

She gave us the "don't stare, but it's okay to glance" talk and showed us the trails, the pool area (bustling), and the clubhouse, which had a game room, bookshelves, and space for karaoke and dances (yes, the night I was there). It was giving off a wholesome, community vibe. I'm talking naked poker, where you *put on* clothes instead of taking them off.

When the tour ended, I filled up my water bottle (all potable water, they have to truck it in), and asked NJ, "So...do I just take my clothes off here?"

"YEP! Anywhere you want!" she said with the enthusiasm of a coach yelling "Go team!"

I drove my car to the hiking trail, stripped naked—except for my socks, shoes, and backpack—and set off. Just your average naked woman with a backpack on a hike.

It was a bit awkward at first, especially since yoga

pants usually shield my legs from every stray branch and blade of grass. I sprayed on natural bug repellent, because if there's one thing I wasn't risking, it's bug bites on bits that are usually covered.

I crossed paths with a friendly 70-ish man sipping on an Emergen-C drink. Two naked strangers, chit-chatting about life. Completely normal, right? (It didn't feel weird with older guys—though I was curious how I'd feel around men closer to my age.) Admittedly at this point, I had some strong dialogue going on in my head. I am literally standing naked with a 70-year-old man, and we are talking about music, hiking trails, and vitamins. Not weird at all in another universe – just not the one I was used to.

After my hike, I decided to join the "cool kids" and head to the pool area. I sprawled out by the pool on a lounge chair. An older gentleman (mid 70s) came by and started setting up a spot for him and wife right next to me. We began chatting. I was on the lounge chair, and he was standing. I was very much respecting the eye contact rule as I was literally at eye level with his dangling bits. In any other scenario, this would be harrowing, but at that moment? Totally normal. After all, we were on Planet Nude. He shared stories about his life, and there we were, without the literal and figurative "clothes" we usually wear in the world. It was oddly liberating.

Later, a younger guy (we'll call him Joseph) sat down a couple chairs away. Joseph was wholesome, handsome, and kind, and he sported an all-American look. He told me he started coming to places like this after visiting a clothing-optional hot springs. His engagement had ended, and his running career changed so he was in the "Embrace Single Me" stage. Another guy joined our conversation (we'll call him Hugh), and shared how he always loved being nude—even as a kid—and found his tribe here. Hugh, by the way, is a successful aerospace engineer.

Joseph invited me to play ping pong. Naked. In what other world is *that* a thing? We crushed it. The game, not the dangly part.

Afterward, I soaked in the hot tub with three people who all had different reasons for embracing nudism. One guy was an art model, another came out as gay and found comfort in his own skin, and one guy's wife, a mother of four, had rediscovered her body here after childbirth.

Joseph, Hugh, and I decided to go on another hike in the woods, this time to a cool chair on a rock. Picture this: three naked people hiking, each staring at the next person's bare butt without a care in the world. For a woman, this setting could be a nightmare or a fantasy (no judgment). But it was...just a hike.

Eventually, we made it to the rock. You had to climb a rope to get to the top of the rock and sit in the chair. So, I climbed up with their encouragement and got to the top of the rock. There I sat on the chair seeing the view of the trees and mountains. It was liberating! I asked Hugh to take a picture of me sitting in the chair. Those pics will probably resurface in 40 years like Rose's naked sketch from *Titanic*. And just like Rose, I will feel bad-ass in my wrinkly skin looking at those photos. Thanks, Hugh.

Six hours had flown by, and it was time to leave. I earned the Naked Badge. I felt freer and braver than ever before.

Now, I know you have questions. I didn't forget. I got your back, fully clothed friends.

Was it hard to not look down at people's parts? You can't help but look. I have never seen that many penisus in my life, all in various sizes, shapes, and colors. And not standing at attention. So yes, you do glance, you just don't stare.

Were you totally naked, or is this more like boobs out, but bottoms on? Totally naked, although some people had open robes on.

Was it cold? If it was cold, I would probably not have done it. But it was a beautiful day with sunshine and gorgeous warm weather.

Was this like a sex party? Quite the opposite. They work hard to create a free yet wholesome environment. This is not Senior Citizens gone wild. I was skeptical about children being allowed, and that was echoed by several friends I told about it before I came. There weren't kids there when I was there. I would say maybe not a great place for teenagers (particularly male teenagers). But for younger kids, it would be fine.

Were there only old people? There was quite a bit of older people there yes. They are currently hoping younger people will start joining to continue the legacy of this place. There were about 30% of people in their 20s and 30s. One guy was tan all over (yes all over) and looked like he was ripped out of a Hercules ad. Ratio-wise, men may have eeked out a few more spots that day, but it didn't feel overly male.

What was the lady's bush levels like? Most were shaved or groomed. Again, I didn't stare so I can't give a full answer to this one.

Did you get any numbers? I kept in touch with my two naked hiking buddies. I even tried to fix Joseph up with one of my twin daughters his same age. But I think it would be weird to see your daughter's boyfriend naked before they do.

Would I do this experience again? I think I would. As a matter of fact, the very next day I went to Desert Reef, a clothing optional hot springs located in Florence, Colorado. This place was located in the middle of nowhere. I drove about two miles down a dirt road until I got to the quaint hots springs area. It reminded me of an area with hot springs in the middle of nowhere as well. It was small, but well done and had 5 pools with varying temperatures to choose from. No phones were allowed, and they encouraged whispering. Most people followed the quiet mode except for a chatty couple (sorry about your custody issues Ted). As far as nudity, about half of the people were in bathing suits, and the rest were either tops off or naked (a big change from the day before). The other interesting part is you can't go there as a man unless you come with a woman. So naturally, there were couples or just women there. It would be a good place to relax at $35 (on the weekends) to go for two and a half hours. MAR is something special though – a great first stop for newbies, and the place I enjoyed most.

Tips if you want to try this:

- Google nude places in your area (or far far far away from your area).
- Bring a robe or cover up for your first time.
- I heard that Orient Land Trust was a really great nude place to go with beautiful gardens.
- Do your research on the resort or location. Not all nudist resorts are created equal. Some are more "family-friendly," while others might have a different vibe. Know what you're getting into so you can feel comfortable and safe.
- Bring a towel. You're going to need it! The number one rule of nudist resorts is: no bare bottoms on communal seats. Whether it's by the pool, in the sauna, or in the lounge, a towel is a must.

UNTITLED

Experience #47: Made Delicious Dairy Magic in a Cheesemaking Class

UNTITLED

Experience #48: Got Up High in a Hot Air Balloon Ride

UNTITLED

Experience #49: Attended a Live TedX Talk

EXPERIENCE #50: WROTE AND PUBLISHED A BOOK

You, my friend, are holding #50.

And what a journey it has been to write this book.

If I haven't said it already, thank you. Thank you for picking up this book (or tablet) and going on each experience with me.

This book started with an idea: try 50 new things. Then I wrote a course called *The Year You Turn 50*. I shared it with no one. Not the most effective way to get it out there, I admit. I decided to share a new #50 experience on my podcast each week, and I was satisfied with doing it that way—until I wasn't. Something was calling me to put this into a book.

Now, I realize there are so many books out there, and the chances of the one you write getting more than a few readers are slim. But I didn't write it for anything more than the experience of having my story down on paper, with the hope of inspiring others. This, to me, is a win! And if nobody reads it but me (and you), it's still a win. We get so caught up sometimes in the end results, the expectations, the "shoulds." The real joy, however, is in the journey.

It took me months to write. I was gung-ho at the beginning, then it went on pause when work got busy. Finally, I committed to writing three chapters every Sunday. Some of the earlier #50 experiences were written right after I had them. Others, I had to relisten to my podcast episodes to relive. My sister, an amazing writer and author herself, was a great resource for bouncing ideas off of and sharing her process when she wrote her book.

About 22 years ago, I wrote a book that I never did anything with. It was written during my religious era about a woman who gets raped and then, through God, finds forgiveness. Except, I had never been raped. The story was fluffy and weak, written in a time when I wasn't living authentically. I found the typed pages in a binder a few months ago while cleaning my garage. I laughed while scanning through it. It was terrible. I had sent it off to a publisher, who rejected it. Thank you, publisher, for small mercies.

This time, I really wanted to produce something I could be proud of sharing. Who knows—will I look back in 20 years and squirm? Maybe. Does it matter? Not really.

Deciding to write was the first step. Doing the writing was harder (but rewarding). The publishing part? That was a whole different experience. My sister shared that she used Atticus (a website and app) to publish her book. It formats the book and makes it easier to convert to e-books and print. So, I wrote my book in Microsoft Word and then brought it over to Atticus for formatting. Once that was completed, I had my sister, a journalist, former editor, and awesome book writer herself, edit the book. I had planned to self-publish on my own until I realized what a huge task that was and the limited time, I had to get this out before the end of 2024.

I interviewed several companies, all with varying degrees of helpfulness and prices. I found the top-rated ones on the Alliance of Independent Authors. You can check out all the ratings here: https://selfpublishingadvice.org/best-self-publishing-services/ They have an excellent review system. The publishing world has some great companies and some scammy ones, and this helped filter it down to my top 15. I had a quick turnaround date (it had to happen before the end of 2024), so some companies were hesitant to say yes. My final top ones after interviewing several were Foglio Print, Aaxek Author Group, and Paperhouse Publishing. I finally decided on Paperhouse because I felt they had the staffing numbers for the quick turnaround, good reviews, and fair market pricing.

There are many companies that specialize in different aspects of the publishing process (like editing), and some do it all. Given my timeline, I chose a company that could help with everything from proofreading the manuscript to getting it published. To give you an idea, my publishing package included full cover design (my Canva design wasn't going to cut it), ISBN (the specific number for your book), copyright protection, layout design for paperback and eBook, interior book formatting, uploading it to a Print on Demand service (like Amazon or IngramSpark), metadata research, bulk printing, and a dedicated project manager. It also stated that I would have 100% rights and royalties. Who knew so much went into getting a book out there! You have my respect, J.K. Rowling and Jane Austen. Extra kudos to Jane, who had to write during a time when women authors weren't prevalent, and computers didn't exist.

Since this book was written in real time, I also knew that I won't be able to comment on what comes after proofreading because it has to end somewhere to actually go to print. If you are wondering how it all works, you can contact one of the publishing companies above, or listen to a great podcast called selfpublishing.com. There are so many great resources out there to help aspiring authors!

I often get asked about the title. It came to me when I decided to visit a nude resort. Yes, it was a bit risqué, but I did, in fact, get naked at 50 (experience #46). More importantly, turning 50 was about embracing the raw, new experiences in life—at an age when many see it as the end of truly living fully.

Would I do this experience again? Maybe. I think if I felt passionately about another topic as I do with this one, I would be open to doing it. It felt great to be writing again as I used to have a blog many years ago.

Tips if you want to try it:

- Write about something you are passionate about (remember-we are living authentically now)
- Use your own voice. Discover what makes your perspective unique. Embrace your own style and let it shine through in your writing to create a voice that stands out. I used AI to edit my book for grammar before handing it over to my sister, and I had to edit AI because it took my voice away. Use it wisely.
- Set realistic goals and break your writing project into manageable chunks. Set achievable daily or weekly word count targets to keep yourself on track and motivated.
- Plan your book's structure before diving in. An outline helps organize your thoughts, maintain focus, and ensure a coherent flow of ideas. If you end up going a different direction, give yourself the grace to do so.
- Establish a regular writing schedule that fits your lifestyle. Consistency helps build momentum and makes the writing process less daunting.
- Understand that your first draft is just the beginning. Be prepared to revise and polish your work through multiple drafts to refine your manuscript and improve clarity.

- If writing is in your heart, go for it! Remember to lean into the experience instead of the end result. They can't all be New York Times Bestsellers, but they can still be something you are passionate about.

EPILOGUE

TO LIVE IS NOT TO SIMPLY BREATHE, BUT TO CHASE THE DREAMS WE DARE TO WEAVE.

WE CAN PLAN A LOT IN LIFE, MOVING FORWARD ON THE PATH we think will last forever. And then life happens. A relationship starts or ends. We lose a loved one. We become a parent. Our jobs change. Our health improves, or our health changes. In May of 2023, our department at work was laid off. Instead of accepting a job offer with the company taking over, I decided to start my own coaching and public speaking business. I knew I was an experienced and qualified coach and speaker, but I didn't know how to run a business. Still, I knew deeply that this was the right choice for me. I released the attachment to it having to work out perfectly or even last forever. I leaned into it with my entire heart (and my very mediocre business acumen).

During this time, I also enrolled in a group coaching program on abundance with Cathy Heller. It was a virtual, three-month program focused on your mindset around possibilities. Again, I let go of expectations. I used savings that I was scared to use to enrolling the course, trusting that the universe would provide the next step on whatever path called to me. I was able to be fully present in this program, and because of that, my mindset opened doors I never could have imagined.

Before I knew it, I was presenting wellness talks to Google and Microsoft (pro bono—but still!). My oldest son, who hadn't been in contact with me for years, called me, and we reconciled, and I joyfully got to go to see him marry his beautiful bride. I wrote two complete courses, gave many free presentations, and kept growing in the process. One day, Cathy Heller shared a podcasting program she was offering. Never did I ever think about creating a podcast. Besides, I was out of funds, so I didn't sign up for this one, but my sister did, as well as some other women I had met in the Abundance course.

Then one day, sort of on an inspired whim, I thought, *Why not do a podcast?* The flow happened so naturally, and again, I had the space and time to do it. So, before I knew it, *Living on the Exhale* was born. At the time of writing this book, I have released over 110 episodes. Will it continue? Will the name change? I don't know. I've let go of what it "has to be" and embraced the journey of creation instead. As someone who writes her goals on a whiteboard every week, letting go of expectations is a big deal for me.

The courses I wrote were bought by only one friend. The coaching program? Two people enrolled. Not very successful by the world's metrics. But oh, the inner growth!

When I started podcasting about my *Year I Turned 50* experiences, I never had a book in mind. Ever. I was just excited to have an intentional year. Then one day in late spring, it came to me that this is what I should do. The courses, the podcasts, and the coaching were all breadcrumbs leading me to this moment of writing a book. Isn't life funny that way? When we let go of what the puzzle should look like and do what lights us up, the pieces appear.

Intentionally seeking new experiences kept me open to saying yes. When I look back at some of them, they were never on my radar! In January 2024, I had zero plans to walk the Camino or even thought riding on a private jet was possible. And yet, here we are.

There were experiences that didn't make it either into the book and/or the podcast. Keeping both zoos and a wildlife retreat seemed like a lot of animal repetition, as did jumping into cold water. Those didn't make the book, but they did make for some great memories. Here are a few:

- Jumping into the freezing ocean with friends in February
- Eating and seeing wild alligators
- Trying out the *Too Good to Go* app

- Going to the Brevard Zoo in Florida, and walking in an open-air area with kangaroos,
- Doing a cold plunge

Looking back now, *Naked at 50* has come to mean more than I ever expected when I first set out on this journey. At 50, I didn't just confront the usual changes that come with age; I peeled away everything that no longer served me—the fears, the doubts, the roles I felt I had to play. I embraced what it meant to live authentically, shedding the need to hide or pretend. And in doing so, I discovered a deeper strength, a confidence that wasn't about appearances, but about owning who I truly am. This journey wasn't just about new experiences; it was about finding joy in living fully and being open to possibility. My hope is that as you've read these pages, you've started to feel a little naked too—ready to shed what's weighing you down and open to embrace your own unfiltered, unapologetic self.

AFFIRMATIONS FOR 50

Let's face it. Sometimes 50 can feel new and exciting. Sometimes it feels like a punch in the stomach. For those days when you need an extra little golden hug, try saying these affirmations.

1. I embrace the wisdom that comes with each passing year.

2. My life is a journey of continuous growth and self-discovery.

3. I am grateful for the experiences that have shaped me into who I am today.

4. I release any fears or doubts about getting older; each year is a gift.

5. I am confident in the knowledge and skills I have acquired over the years.

6. My age is a testament to the resilience and strength within me.

7. I celebrate the milestones of my past and look forward to new adventures ahead.

8. I am surrounded by love, joy, and positive energy.

9. I trust the path that has led me to this point and the journey that lies ahead.

10. Every day is an opportunity for me to learn, grow, and thrive.

11. I am a source of inspiration for others as I embrace my true self.

12. I am at peace with my past and excited about the possibilities of my future.

13. The best is yet to come, and I welcome it with open arms.

14. I am a beacon of wisdom, grace, and authenticity.

15. I am grateful for the lessons learned and the strength gained from challenges.

16. My age is not a limitation but a source of empowerment.

17. I radiate confidence, self-love, and positive energy.

18. I am in tune with my body, mind, and spirit, creating a harmonious balance.

19. I attract abundance and prosperity into my life effortlessly.

20. Each day, I choose joy, gratitude, and love.

21. I am proud of the person I have become and the values I uphold.

22. My life is a beautiful tapestry of experiences, woven with love and resilience.

23. I honor the past, live in the present, and eagerly anticipate the future.

24. I am surrounded by supportive relationships that uplift and inspire me.

25. I am open to new adventures and embrace the opportunities that come my way.

26. My age is a reflection of the countless blessings in my life.

27. I release the need for perfection and accept myself as a work in progress.

28. I am a wise and capable individual, capable of achieving my goals.

29. I am deserving of love, respect, and all the good things life has to offer.

30. I radiate vitality, strength, and positive energy.

31. I trust in the wisdom of my body and treat it with love and care.

32. I am a beacon of light, bringing positivity to every situation.

33. I am surrounded by supportive friends and family who cherish and celebrate me.

34. I let go of anything that no longer serves my highest good.

35. I am an inspiration to those around me, leaving a positive impact.

36. I am at ease with the aging process and embrace the beauty it brings.

37. My experiences have made me resilient, wise, and compassionate.

38. I am open to receiving the abundance that the universe has in store for me.

39. I am an important and valuable member of my community.

40. My life is a reflection of the love and kindness I've

shared with others.

41. I trust in the divine timing of my life's journey.

42. I am a beacon of wisdom, compassion, and joy.

43. I radiate confidence and grace in every situation.

44. I am a magnet for positive opportunities and experiences.

45. I am proud of my accomplishments and excited about what's yet to come.

46. I embrace change as a natural and necessary part of life.

47. I am a source of inspiration, strength, and encouragement for others.

48. I am surrounded by beauty, love, and abundance.

49. I am the architect of my life, and I build its foundation with gratitude and joy.

50. I celebrate the incredible journey of my life and look forward to the adventures ahead.

ACKNOWLEDGMENTS

The acknowledgements page is a place to say thank you to anyone or anything who has helped make the book possible. Being a part of the back matter, authors will often use acknowledgements to recognize a number of sources, or offer more detail about why the source is being recognized.

PART TWO
LOOKING BACK

PART THREE
LOOKING FORWARD

UNTITLED

Stay in Touch

Made in the USA
Las Vegas, NV
12 November 2024

11648402R00197